NURSING THEORIES

The Base for Professional Nursing Practice

The Nursing Theories Conference Group

Julia B. George, Chairperson

PRENTICE-HALL, INC., Englewood Cliffs, New Jersey 07632

Library of Congress Cataloging in Publication Data

NURSING THEORIES CONFERENCE GROUP.
  Nursing theories.

  Includes bibliographical references and index.
  1. Nursing–Philosophy. I. George, Julia B.
II. Title.
RT84.5.N88 1980   610.73'01   79-15063
ISBN 0-13-627703-9

Editorial/production supervision
  and interior design: Eleanor Henshaw Hiatt
Cover design: Wanda Lubelska
Manufacturing buyer: Cathie Lenard

Printed in the United States of America

10 9 8 7

PRENTICE-HALL INTERNATIONAL, INC., *London*
PRENTICE-HALL OF AUSTRALIA PTY. LIMITED, *Sydney*
PRENTICE-HALL OF CANADA, LTD., *Toronto*
PRENTICE-HALL OF INDIA PRIVATE LIMITED, *New Delhi*
PRENTICE-HALL OF JAPAN, INC., *Tokyo*
PRENTICE-HALL OF SOUTHEAST ASIA PTE. LTD., *Singapore*
WHITEHALL BOOKS LIMITED, *Wellington, New Zealand*

CONTRIBUTING AUTHORS

Janice Ryan Belcher, R.N., M.S., Instructor, School of Nursing, Wright State University, Dayton, Ohio

Agnes M. Bennett, R.N., M.S.N., Assistant Professor, School of Nursing, Wright State University, Dayton, Ohio

Mary Disbrow Crane, R.N., M.S., Assistant Professor, School of Nursing, University of Evansville, Evansville, Indiana

Connie Hetrick Esposito, R.N., M.S.N., Assistant Professor, School of Nursing, Wright State University, Dayton, Ohio

Suzanne M. Falco, R.N., Ph.D., Associate Professor and Assistant Dean, School of Nursing, Wright State University, Dayton, Ohio

Lois J. Brittain Fish, R.N., M.S.N., Assistant Director of Nursing/Nursing Education, The Children's Medical Center, Dayton, Ohio

Peggy Coldwell Foster, R.N., M.S.N., Former Instructor, School of Nursing, Wright State University, Dayton, Ohio

Chiyoko Yamamoto Furukawa, R.N., M.S., Visiting Assistant Professor, College of Nursing, University of New Mexico, Albuquerque, New Mexico

Julia Gallagher Galbreath, R.N., M.S., Instructor, School of Nursing, Wright State University, Dayton, Ohio

Julia B. George, R.N., M.S., Assistant Professor, School of Nursing, Wright State University, Dayton, Ohio

Kathleen Hale, R.N., M.S., Instructor, Hunter College, New York, New York

Joan K. Howe, R.N., M.S., Former Assistant Professor, School of Nursing, Wright State University, Dayton, Ohio

Nancy P. Janssens, R.N., M.S., Director, Continuing Education, School of Nursing, Wright State University, Dayton, Ohio

Mary Kathryn Leonard, R.N., M.S., Assistant Professor, School of Nursing, Wright State University, Dayton, Ohio

Marie L. Lobo, R.N., M.N., Predoctoral student, Nursing Science, University of Washington, Seattle, Washington; Former Assistant Professor, School of Nursing, Wright State University, Dayton, Ohio

Charlotte Paul, R.N., Ph.D., Former Assistant Professor, School of Nursing, Wright State University, Dayton, Ohio

Joan S. Reeves, R.N., M.S.N., Former Instructor, School of Nursing, Wright State University, Dayton, Ohio

Marjorie Stanton, R.N., Ed.D., Professor and Associate Dean, School of Nursing, Wright State University, Dayton, Ohio

Gertrude Torres, R.N., Ed.D., Professor and Dean, School of Nursing, Wright State University, Dayton, Ohio

CONTENTS

v

PREFACE

Nursing is an increasingly emerging profession. As such, it is deeply involved in identifying its own unique knowledge base. In identifying this base of knowledge, concepts and theories specific to nursing are being developed and recognized. Over the years several individuals have promoted a concept or theory of nursing. Although these various concepts/theories have been published in a variety of journals and books, they have never been gathered in one volume and applied to nursing practice through the nursing process.

This book is designed to consider the ideas of twelve nursing theorists and relate the work of each to the nursing process of assessing, diagnosing, planning, implementing, and evaluating. The book is intended for use as a tool for the application of nursing concepts and theories to nursing practice.

There are essentially three areas of focus. Chapters 1 and 2 present the place of concepts and theories in nursing and discuss the nursing process. These chapters provide a common base for the next twelve chapters and should be read first. Chapters 3 through 14 present the major components of the work of Florence Nightingale, Lydia E. Hall, Virginia Henderson, Hildegard E. Peplau, Dorothea E. Orem, Faye G. Abdellah, Ida Jean Orlando, Ernestine Wiedenbach, Myra Estrin Levine, Martha E. Rogers, Imogene M. King, and Sister

Callista Roy. Each of these chapters presents one theorist and may be read in any order. The chapter contents give the historical setting of the nursing theorist and the specific components that she identified as meaningful to nursing. This material is drawn from the work of each theorist. The components are then interpreted and discussed by the chapter author(s) in relation to the four basic concepts of man, health, society, and nursing and to their use in the nursing process. Chapter 15 is an aid to the reader for using several to all the theories presented in the nursing process in a given situation. This last chapter presents some examples of application of the components as a guide and stimulus to the reader's thought processes and utilization of theory and the nursing process for professional nursing practice. Chapter 15 will be most meaningful if it is read after becoming familiar with the contents of Chapters 1 through 14.

The term *man*, when used as one of the four basic concepts, (man, health, society, and nursing), is used in the generic sense to include persons of all ages and sexes. Some of the theorists, as appropriate to their times, used *she* to refer to the nurse and *he* to refer to the recipient of care. In some chapters it would have been awkward to change the theorist's use of such words. In these situations, we have indicated that the use is that of the original author. In all other cases, we have used the generic meaning of man.

The Nursing Theories Conference Group was formed out of a concern for the need for materials to help students of nursing understand and use nursing theories in nursing practice. The original group of ten nursing faculty members began discussions in 1975. The need for a text that included the elements of various nursing theories and their application to practice soon became apparent. As the theories to be included were identified, the group gradually expanded to include the nineteen contributing authors of this book. All the contributing authors have at some time been associated with Wright State University School of Nursing. It was this proximity that led to their membership in the Group. Although membership in The Nursing Theories Conference Group is likely to keep changing, the Group will continue its efforts to enhance the development of theory-based professional nursing practice.

Suggestions and comments from users of this text are welcome.

Julia B. George
Chairperson,
The Nursing Theories Conference Group

1

THE PLACE OF CONCEPTS
AND THEORIES WITHIN NURSING

Gertrude Torres

Basic to any professional discipline is the development of a body of knowledge that can be applied to its practice. Such knowledge is often expressed in terms of concepts and theories, especially in the area of the behavioral or social sciences. Thus, nursing as a young, evolving profession is beginning to develop a body of knowledge in terms of the concepts and theories that support its practice.

The use and meanings of the terms *concept* and *theory* within nursing and other disciplines are often conflicting. This confusion can be caused by differences of opinion. However, such confusion is more likely to be caused by the frequent use of these terms in a broad nondefined sense, leaving the listeners or readers uncertain as to the purpose of the presentation and encouraging them to focus on details or specifics rather than on concepts.

In 1920, Lavinia Dock and I.M. Stewart, in discussing the education of nursing for the future, stated that the *concept* of public health and the normal healthy individual should be taught before the care of the sick individual. Although they did not define what was meant by *concept*, one can conjecture that the term was used because they apparently viewed public health as a concept.[1]

In 1933, the New York League of Nursing Education prepared a *concept* of nursing that defined nursing as "using skillfully scientific methods in adapting prescribed therapy and preventive treatment to the specific physical and psychic needs of the individual."[2] A year later in the *American Journal of Nursing*, Effie Taylor spoke of the prevailing concept of nursing as practical, having real depths through love, sympathy, knowledge, and culture.[3] In 1969, Faye Abdellah proposed that nursing theories are the basis for nursing sciences. Among those she identified as being pioneers in the development of nursing theories were Ida Jean Orlando, Ernestine Wiedenbach, and Hildegard Peplau.[4]

The use of the word *concept* is not a new phenomenon; it is one that has been part of nursing's historical background. This is also probably true in other disciplines within and outside the health care fields. Nursing has used the word *concept* for over fifty years without its having a specific meaning and will probably continue to do so for several more decades.

The main purpose of this chapter is to present the various approaches to the meanings of the words *concept* and *theory* and to identify each definition that is functional and should be applied in reading this book.

Concepts are basically vehicles of thought that involve images.[5] They are abstract notions and are similar in definition to ideas.[6] Impressions received by sensing our environment evolve into concepts.[7] Individuals vary in the specific images or notions they perceive in relation to a given concept. In nursing, the most significant concepts that influence and determine its practice are man, society, health, and nursing (see Figure 1-1). Among these four concepts, the core of the practice of nursing is man. It is from the client or patient that the other nursing concepts arise. Without any of these concepts, nursing cannot evolve either as a science or as a professional practice field. For example, nursing and man may have little relationship unless one recognizes some aspect of health, such as its promotion or restoration, as part of a mutual concern. Also, to attempt to envision man without a society significantly tests one's thought processes.

Since specific concepts create images abstract in nature, these concepts tend to have different meanings and they lead to individual interpretations. They are strongly influenced by previous learning experiences. Thus, the concept of man creates an almost endless supply of notions and ideas. For example, the concept of man creates images related to woman, soldier, patient, human being, father, son, and so forth. This kind of word association also leads to identifying related

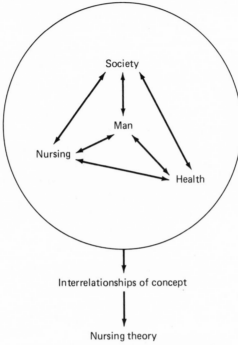

Interrelationships of concept

Nursing theory

Figure 1-1. Concepts essential to practice.

concepts so that increased clarification can occur. In communicating, individuals often use concepts followed by some explanation or description in order to increase the clarity of the message. Misinterpretation, which can lead to misunderstanding, is caused by lack of clarification in the meaning of words as concepts. It is not essential to agree on the meaning of a particular concept, but it is important to describe it sufficiently so that the image one attempts to project becomes less abstract. Undefined concepts tend to be too generalized in nature to assist in understanding specifics, and defined concepts do not necessarily indicate a plan for implementation. For this reason, the use of concepts alone without theories is of little assistance in influencing nursing practice.

If nursing accepts the idea that concepts are the elements used to develop theories, which form the basis for nursing practice, the profession must then have a thorough understanding of the meaning of the word *theory*.

Within nursing and many disciplines the meaning of the word *theory* varies. Nursing needs to recognize that this variety of interpretations is a method of searching and exploring for truths and clarity.

Although the lack of precise definition may lead some to a state of confusion and frustration, it allows the option of developing a definition of *theory* that is functional for nursing practice. As the nursing profession matures, sophistication in the understanding and utilizing of nursing theories will probably increase.

In order to give some clarity to the word *theory* so that it can be functional throughout this book, a review of some of the literature is necessary. The word evolves from the Greek word *theoria* signifying a "vision." Rather than sensory in nature, the development of theories should be viewed as rational and intellectual and leading to the disclosure of truth. Involved in this intellectual process is comparing, experimenting, and uncovering relationships.[8] This approach to the meaning of theory makes most individuals in nursing potential theory builders. Thus, it is important that nursing recognize that anyone who is capable of speaking is a potential theorist. Nursing frequently claims to have visions or truths about beliefs that strongly influence actions. Although this interpretation is helpful in allowing the profession to believe that anyone is capable of theorizing as an intellectual human being, it is of little true value in the development of a sound body of knowledge based on research derived from theory. Theories need to do more than foster intellectual visions on how nurses might practice.

Theories are also viewed as a set of interrelated concepts that give a systematic view of a phenomenon that is explanatory and predictive in nature.[9] Ideally, nursing theories should be viewed as an interrelationship of these basic concepts and should be used to systematically explain approaches to nursing care and to predict outcomes. The extent of predictability depends on the amount of research available and on the theorist's skill in studying the research and in linking concepts and theories to form new theories. Nurses all too frequently use intuition, habit, or tradition as the basis for making nursing decisions. For example, in caring for a client/patient with a particular need/problem, using a particular nursing theory should give strong clues as to the outcomes of nursing care. If one relates this to the use of a particular drug, given the correct data about a patient/client and the drug, one expects certain results to occur from the administration of that drug. Thus, the outcome has the element of prediction. This approach to the meaning of theory is a rather sophisticated one for nursing at the present time. Those in nursing should view a theory as a way of relating concepts through the use of definitions that assist in developing significant interrelationships to describe or classify approaches to practice (see Figure 1-1). Classification can be used to relate facts and to generalize about homogeneous groups. This will assist in explaining events.[10] Although this approach does not provide the important predictive ingredient of a theory, it does permit viewing nursing theories as a way of assisting and explaining approaches to practice.

In other fields, especially the biological sciences, there are principles and laws as well as theories. Laws and principles are truly *predictable* and can be utilized with assurance because they provide a sound body of knowledge in which to function. For example, in chemistry, if one correctly places a salt and an acid in the same vehicle, one can predict the results. Laws, principles, and theories derived from laws and principles compose the basis for the pure sciences. On the other hand, since nursing is similar to the behavioral sciences, its knowledge for nursing practice is primarily based on theories. In the future, the predictability of nursing theories will become more reliable as concepts are better defined and as the research base from which theories develop grows.

Theories are a way of combining concepts for the purpose of deriving hypotheses about practice. In reviewing theories, it is important to understand their basic characteristics. These are reviewed below.

THE BASIC CHARACTERISTICS OF THEORIES

Theories can interrelate concepts in such a way as to create a different way of looking at a particular phenomenon. When significant relationships are identified between the concepts of man and nursing, such relationships can be viewed in a more defined manner. The concepts of man and nursing as abstract notions are too broad and too generalized by themselves. But describing and explaining the relationships of the two concepts can create a new way of understanding them. If man is viewed as having needs and nursing as having the function of providing these needs, a relationship that connects these concepts is found. Again, the concepts of man, health, and nursing can be related by hypothesizing that nursing as a practice discipline deals and interacts with man in relation to man's state of well-being. Here man is conceptualized as interactive, health as a state of well-being, and nursing as a practice discipline. Adding the concept of society to the previous relationship, one can then view society as involving families as well as individuals who interact with nursing in relation to their state of well-being. The greater the scope of the relationships, the more significant the theory is likely to be.

Theories must be logical in nature.   Logic involves orderly reasoning. Interrelationships must be sequential and must follow principles of reasoning. In order to use theories, these theories must be logical in their propositions so that contradictions are not apparent. One should be able to use the theory in a reasonable manner to explain the consequences of actions.

Theories can be the bases for hypotheses that can be tested.   If a particular theory cannot be tested, it offers little as a base of knowledge. The theory should be sufficiently understandable so that hypotheses can be developed that can be tested. Reliability of prediction increases when retesting in a similar situation shows the same conclusions. It is through this validation that the theory grows in meaning and significance.

Theories contribute to and assist in increasing the general body of knowledge within the discipline through the research implemented to validate them.   Further validation of theories through researching hypotheses derived from them not only contributes to the present body of knowledge but leads to the development of other scientific theories from which hypotheses can be drawn. Thus theories, if sound, assist in developing nursing hypotheses that can be used to develop new theories.

Theories can be utilized by the practitioners to guide and improve their practice.   The most significant characteristic of a theory is its usefulness to the practitioner. Although nursing theories presently do not predict outcomes, they are very helpful in providing practitioners with guidelines to test and validate their approaches to nursing care. The essence of a professional is to use the theories of the discipline to practice his profession.

Theories must be consistent with other validated theories, laws, and principles. Unless nursing theories build upon scientific findings that have been validated, much confusion will occur. Since nursing practice is based on a scientific and humanitarian foundation, any nursing theory must support such knowledge. As the various nursing theories are presented throughout the text, comparisons should be made between previously learned theories and these new nursing theories.

By examining the following situation, one can identify how a theoretical approach can be utilized in nursing practice.

Situation. Mrs. Mary Dolphin is nine months pregnant and is expecting her first child within a week. She is visiting her obstetrician for an examination. The office nurse has been requested to do health teaching either during the office visits or in Mrs. Dolphin's home. Mrs. Dolphin is an executive career woman of Irish descent who has been married for one year. Mr. Dolphin is in governmental service and travels a great deal, frequently leaving Mrs. Dolphin alone. During the entire pregnancy, Mrs. Dolphin has been cooperative and enthusiastic. No complications or unusual problems (other than morning sickness, which lasted for six weeks during her first trimester) have occurred during the pregnancy.

In reviewing the above situation, many theories, especially those related to the sciences, can be identified that would show the need of special knowledge in order to practice professional nursing. The following kinds of theories reflect only a sample.

KINDS OF THEORIES

Stress Theories

The nurse needs to assess the patient's previous ability to deal with stress. Theories that give clues as to how man deals physiologically and psychologically with stress will assist the nurse in understanding how patients/clients can be expected to react. Stress theories will also enable the nurse to differentiate between typical and atypical reactions to stress, thus leading to more appropriate nursing diagnoses.

Developmental Theories

Theories relating to the development of each member of the family will give the nurse an appropriate knowledge base on which to assess specific developmental levels and tasks for each member of the family. For example, during Mrs. Dolphin's pregnancy, it is important for the nurse to teach her what is the "normal" physical, intellectual, and emotional development of the newborn and the infant, as well as the "normal" development of the pregnant family.

Family Theories

The structure and function of the family unit and the interrelationships of a family group are reflected in theories relating to the family. Although the office nurse may not have seen Mr. Dolphin, the nurse is able to assess Mrs. Dolphin's relationship with her husband as perceived by Mrs. Dolphin and the impact that a new child may have on the family relationships. Theories concerning family structure and needs will assist the professional nurse in health teaching and nursing diagnoses.

Interactive Theories

The professional nurse must have a sound base of theoretical knowledge about interactions since the base of health teaching relates to the nurse's ability to interact with Mrs. Dolphin and Mrs. Dolphin's ability to interact with others.

Adaptation Theories

Mrs. Dolphin needs to be assessed in terms of her ability to adapt to both her pregnancy and the birth of a child. The nurse needs to be able to explain and hypothesize physical and emotional changes in Mrs. Dolphin.

Other theories can also be identified that will offer the nurse insight into both assessing and planning care. For example, *role* theories will assist in explaining both the role of the nurse and the client's role as a mother. *Change* theories will offer insight into the expected behaviors that evolve when significant change occurs within an environment. *Nursing* theories that explain phenomena and guide the nurse in giving care would be instrumental as guidelines to care. It is recognized that nursing theories that are predictive would be the most functional tools to teach and use in nursing practice, but nursing must be content with explanations until predictive theories are developed through increased research. Also, involved in the care of Mrs. Dolphin are a variety of scientific principles related to physiology, such as fetal nourishment, labor, and delivery.

In caring for Mrs. Dolphin, the nurse needs a breadth of knowledge. The greater the nurse's sophistication and expertise in theories, the greater the potential for the utilization of appropriate approaches to care. A strong theoretical knowledge base assists the nurse in providing quality nursing care.

Figure 1-2 gives us a visual reference point by which to identify how theories assist the nurse in the care of Mrs. Dolphin. The reader needs to identify other theories that he or she believes would be essential knowledge bases upon which to provide care for Mrs. Dolphin. A beginning student in nursing should review theories offered in his/her courses that are foundational to nursing.

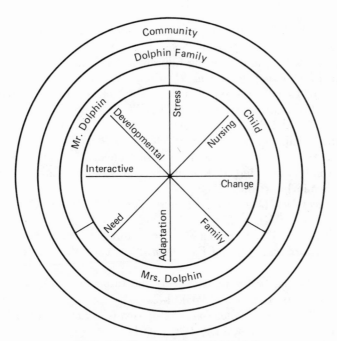

Figure 1-2. Theories—Base of knowledge.

SUMMARY

Concepts represent abstract notions and ideas that, when interrelated, provide the foundation of a theory. Theories may be viewed as visions giving intellectual insight into phenomena, but for maximum significance and impact they should be explanatory and predictive in nature so as to achieve professional practice. Nursing theories need to be viewed in the context of how they describe or classify approaches to practice by interrelating concepts of man, society, health, and nursing. Nursing research through testing hypotheses derived from theories and through assisting in the development of more predictive theories will thereby build a body of nursing science.

Within any given nursing situation, a variety of theories can be identified that will give the professional nurse a strong base of knowledge on which to practice and explain his/her approach to nursing care. The main function of this text is to demonstrate how nursing theories provide this knowledge base for professional nursing practice and ultimately for improving health care.

NOTES

1. Lavinia L. Dock and I. M. Stewart, A Short History of Nursing, 4th ed. (New York: G. P. Putnam's Sons, 1920), p. 249.
2. New York League of Nursing Education, "A Concept of Nursing," The American Journal of Nursing, 33 (June 1933), 565.
3. Effie J. Taylor, "Of What Is the Nature of Nursing?" The American Journal of Nursing, 34 (May 1934), 476.
4. Faye G. Abdellah, "The Nature of Nursing Science," Nursing Research, xviii, no. 5 (September/October 1969), 390.
5. Rom Harre, "The Formal Analysis of Concepts," Analysis of Concept Learning, eds. Herbert Klausmerer and Chester Harris (New York: Academic Press, Inc., 1966), 3–4.
6. Webster's New Collegiate Dictionary (Springfield, Mass.: G. & C. Merriam Co., 1974), p. 233.
7. A. Toffler, "The Psychology of the Future," Learning for Tomorrow— The Role of the Future in Education (New York: Vintage Books, 1974), p. 12.
8. P. H. Phenix, "Educational Theory and Inspiration," Educational Theory, xiii, no. 1 (January 1963), 1–2.
9. F. N. Kerlinger, Foundations of Behavioral Research (New York: Holt, Rinehart & Winston, Inc., 1965), p. 11.
10. G. Beauchamp, Curriculum Theory, 2nd ed. (Wilmette, Ill.: Kagg Press, 1968), pp. 23–24.

2

AN OVERVIEW
OF THE NURSING PROCESS

Marjorie Stanton, Charlotte Paul, and Joan S. Reeves

This chapter is based on the assumption that professional nursing practice is interpersonal in nature. Recognizing the importance and effect of the nurse's relationship with the client/patient, professional nurses use this knowledge in proceeding through each phase of the nursing process.

It is also assumed that professional nurses view human beings as holistic, thereby acknowledging that mind and body are not separate but function as a whole. People respond as whole beings. What happens in one part of the mind or body affects the person as a whole entity.

Given these two assumptions, it would be impossible for a nurse to view a client/patient as "the hysterectomy in room 201" or the "paranoid in bed 2." The woman who has experienced a hysterectomy may have physiological, spiritual, and psychological health problems; i.e., physiological and psychological adjustments due to induced menopause, and spiritual adjustments if her life style included a religious orientation related to a life of childbearing. The person with symptoms of paranoia may refuse to eat, causing physiological changes related to malnutrition. These two assumptions, that nursing is interpersonal in nature and that professional nurses view human beings as holistic, give guidance and direction to the use of the nursing process.

The nursing process is the underlying scheme that provides order and direction to nursing care. It is the essence of professional nursing practice. It is the "tool" and methodology of the nursing profession and, as such, helps nurses in arriving at decisions and in predicting and evaluating consequences. The nursing process can be defined as a deliberate intellectual activity whereby the practice of nursing is approached in an orderly, systematic manner. Each of these terms for defining the process can be further delineated as follows:*

Deliberate: Careful, thoughtful, intentional.

Intellectual: Rational, knowledgeable, reasonable, conceptual.

Activity: The state or condition of functioning, initiating, changing, behaving.

Orderly: A methodical, efficient, logical arrangement.

Systematic: Purposeful, pertaining to classification.

Students of nursing using the nursing process are learning to behave as professional nurses in practice behave. Since the nursing process is the essence and tool (methodology) of professional nursing practice, students must become familiar with and adept at using the nursing process as their basis for practice. The nursing process also provides a means for evaluating the quality of nursing care given by nurses and assures their accountability and responsibility to the client/patient. In order to use the nursing process effectively, nurses need to understand and apply appropriate concepts and theories from nursing, from the biological, physical, and behavioral sciences, and from the humanities, in order to provide a rationale for decision making, judgments, interpersonal relationships, and actions. These concepts and theories provide the framework for nursing care.

FIVE PHASES

Most authors agree that four phases are considered necessary to the nursing process: assessment, nursing diagnosis or identification of problem, intervention or implementation, and evaluation.[1,2,3,4] Some authors do not mention the nursing diagnosis as such, and some consider the nursing care plan separately. However, in this book,

---

*The list is based on definitions found in the *American Heritage Dictionary,* 1975.

because nursing diagnosis is considered an essential component of the nursing process and planning is included as an integral part of the process, the components are as follows:

1. assessment
2. nursing diagnosis
3. planning
4. implementation
5. evaluation

Although this listing of the components suggests a forward movement of the process through each discrete phase, this does not always occur in the actual process. Assessment must always begin the process, and it always leads to a nursing diagnosis. The assessment phase includes collection and analysis of data. The nursing diagnosis derives from assessment. However, during the planning, implementation, and evaluation phases, *reassessment* (the further collection and analysis of data) can lead to immediate changes in each of these three stages before moving on to the next one. Reassessment may also lead to a change in diagnosis, which leads to a change in planning, implementation, and evaluation as the process continues (see Figure 2-1).

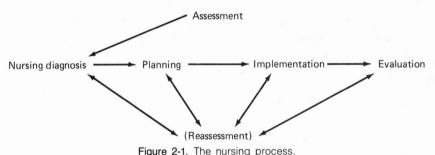

Figure 2-1. The nursing process.

Assessment

Assessment is the first phase in the nursing process. It consists of the systematic and orderly collection and analysis of data pertaining to and about the health status of the client/patient for the purpose of making the nursing diagnosis. It always leads to a nursing diagnosis. Insufficient or incorrect assessment can lead to an incorrect nursing diagnosis, which could mean inappropriate planning, implementation, and evaluation. Therefore, the importance of accurate assessment cannot be overemphasized. It is vital to the process and is the basis for all other stages in the process. Although assessment is the first phase, it may also occur as reassessment during any other phase of the process, except the diagnosis phase, when new data about the client/patient are obtained.[5]

The systematic and orderly collection of data is essential in order for the nurse to know if all possible data have been collected, and it serves to provide a method of quick retrieval of information relative to the client/patient for auditing professional practice and for doing nursing research. Several authors have provided guidelines for the systematic collection of data.[6,7,8,9] The American Nurses' Association's (ANA) *Standards of Nursing Practice* also provides information.[10] A holistic view during the assessment phase insures that the biological, psychological, social, and spiritual spheres of the individual are considered. Any assessment guidelines should include the following:

Biographical data.

A health history including family and social history.

Subjective and objective data about the current health status, including reasons for contact with health care professional and medical diagnosis if the client/patient has a medical problem.

By using these guidelines, the data collected are classified into discrete areas that can be compared and contrasted for relationships during the analysis of the data.

Situation.   Mrs. James has come to the outpatient department medical clinic because "I just don't feel well." Her medical diagnosis is general malaise. An excerpt of the assessment data collected by the nurse for Mrs. James might look like Table 2-1.

The biographical data are generally provided during an interview with the client or the person responsible for the client.[11] Such data are necessary to appropriately identify the client as an individual and may provide clues to the client's health status. For example, the age of clients gives an indication of their growth and developmental status.

A health history is "the client's story of past and present events which may affect current and future health status."[12] The history is obtained through interviewing the client and/or individual responsible for the client, i.e., parent, and by reviewing previous health records of the client if available. Clients may, if able, fill out part of the biographical data and health history forms.

Table 2-1

Assessment of Mrs. James

Bio Data	Health History	Subjective Data	Objective Data
Client—Mary James	Italian/Spanish heritage.	"Fingernails break easily."	Height—5'2" Weight—180 lb.
Age—45 Housewife	Mother of Mrs. James had diabetes in older years.	Favorite foods are pizza, pasta with butter, french fries,	Skin pale, dry to touch. Hair lifeless and
Husband— Philip	"All family are overweight."	biscuits with gravy. Drinks are coffee	dry to touch. Nails are rag-
Age—46 Electrical helper	Shops at local fast-food market.	and Tab. Dislikes milk, meats,	ged and broken.
Daughters— Ann, age—18 Jean, age—15	Usually shops daily. Mrs. James responsible for cooking. Family does not have regular mealtimes.	and vegetables.	

The current health status of the client is ascertained through interviewing the client or person responsible for the client (subjective data) and through examination and observation of the client to obtain data that can be seen or measured objectively (objective data). A client's description of pain is considered to be subjective data. Vital signs are an example of an objective measurement of physiological data.[13] When possible, objective data should be obtained to verify subjective data. For example, the client complains of abdominal pain (subjective data), which the nurse verifies by observation of the position of the client and palpation of the abdomen for tenderness and/or rigidity (objective data).

After the data are collected and classified, analysis of the data takes place. This is the professional nurse's responsibility and *must* occur in order to make a nursing diagnosis. The nurse examines the data to identify, compare, and contrast the relationship of one piece of data to another. The new data collected are also compared to societal norms to identify an actual or potential health problem. For example, a four-year-old who is unable to walk does not meet the developmental standards for four-year-olds, and this is an example of an actual health problem.

The comparison and relationship of data in Table 2-2 indicate that the client may have a potential health problem in relation to diabetes based on age, family history of diabetes, and obesity problem.

It is during the analysis stage of assessment that the nurse uses her knowledge of various theories and concepts to categorize and

Table 2-2

Comparison and Relationship of Data
for Mrs. James

Biographical Data	Health History	Current Health Status
45 years old	Mother had adult onset diabetes	Height—5'2" Weight—180 lbs

classify the data collected. When analyzing the data related to age, the nurse needs to know what is expected of people during each stage of development. Abraham Maslow's hierarchy of needs,[14] E. H. Erikson's eight stages of man,[15] and other sources in the literature are useful references to consider in looking at the data.

Identification of gaps in the data should occur during the analysis stage in order to insure that all important information has been supplied and that the nursing diagnosis is based on actual data and not on inaccurate assumptions. Assessing a young child without talking to the mother or to the person responsible for the child will immediately tell the nurse that there are gaps in the data. An analysis of the data should also give clues as to the kinds of patterns developing. In the case of Mrs. James, there is a pattern of poor eating habits, poor selection of foods, and little understanding of diet for good health. These patterns may be handed down from generation to generation.

Nursing Diagnosis

Nursing diagnosis is the second phase in the nursing process. It is a summary statement describing the client's actual or potential health problems or deficits, based on the nurse's judgment after gathering and analyzing pertinent data.[16] The diagnosis focuses attention on the clients' responses to their health status, life experiences, and coping patterns. The *actual* health problem is that area of concern that is in existence now. It may be a symptom; a physiological finding; or a behavioral, psychosocial, and/or spiritual problem that is an independent nursing concern and is stated as a nursing diagnosis. In the case of Mrs. James, one nursing diagnosis based on the assessment above is: lack of understanding of the basic four food groups and their relationship to health. The potential health problem is identified in the nursing diagnosis statement as being potential. For example, the hazards of immobility associated with a client who is on bed rest may create a potential health problem related to impaired circulation.

As one proceeds through the analysis of the data, certain patterns develop, and the utilization of relevant nursing concepts and theories is appropriate. Gradually the actual nursing diagnosis is formulated, and a statement of conclusion is established. The nursing diagnosis establishes a point from which nursing care can begin and is a means by which statements are formulated about pertinent data obtained in the nursing assessment. It is important to rank or prioritize these nursing diagnoses if there is more than one. One needs to deal with those areas that have the greatest impact on the client and/or family. This ranking should take into consideration both the client's and the nurse's opinion. The nurse also determines priorities based on past nursing experiences and on scientific knowledge of the needs and functions of human beings. Therefore, a continuum of priorities of nursing diagnoses is developed.

When establishing nursing diagnoses and nursing actions, it is important to recognize there are possible consequences that can develop from these actions. Also, there are some factors that may have an effect on the ranking of nursing diagnoses. External factors such as personnel, time, money, prognosis, availability of agencies, agency policies, and the individual value systems of the persons involved may lead to conflicting priorities. These factors must be dealt with on a continuous basis, so the whole system (individual, family, community) can be brought into balance. After nursing diagnoses are established, then the plan for implementation is formulated.

Planning

Planning is the third phase. The plan for providing nursing care can be stated as the determination of what can be done to assist the client, and this involves setting goals and objectives, judging priorities, and designing methods to resolve problems.[17] The first stage in the planning is setting goals and objectives. These goals and objectives are derived from the nursing diagnoses and are established for each nursing diagnosis listed.

In preparing to write the plan, the client and his family should be consulted before formulating the goals and objectives. The goals and objectives should be realistic and attainable, supportive of the client's needs, and mutually acceptable. It is important to consider the need for objectives that can be defined and stated concisely in an "act-of-being" phrase. This phrase should contain a performer (the client), a performance (action), and a change in behavior to be accomplished (objectives). The expected end behavior needs to be identified and be placed in the proper time frame, and can be utilized as a means for evaluation.

Goals are stated in broad terms in order to identify effective criteria for evaluating nursing action. These goals can pertain to rehabilitation, prevention of complications associated with stressors, and/or the ability of the client to adapt to these stressors. Other goals may deal with the achievement of the highest potential for wholeness of the system. A sample of a goal statement would be, "Mrs. James will have an adequate understanding of the basic food groups and their relationship to recommended daily allowance (RDA) requirements within one month."

From the goals, objectives are determined that need to be stated in observable behavioral terms. Objectives should define the conditions under which the expected end behaviors are expected to occur and should specify the acceptable performance level and the specific behaviors that will be accepted as being evidence of meeting the desired outcomes. The behaviors in question refer to psychological, physiological, social, and intellectual activities and other observable responses. Objectives related to the above goal for Mrs. James could be:

1. Identify the basic four food groups from a chart.
2. Prepare a shopping list to include at least two necessary foods from each group by the end of Week I.
3. Prepare family menus for three days using the basic four food groups as a guide by Week II.
4. Make substitutions in family menus for three days using the basic four food groups chart as guide by Week III.
5. Evaluate eating patterns of family for one week using the basic four food groups chart as guide and identify at least two problem areas to discuss with nurse by Week IV.

Desired behavioral outcomes (objectives) should be stated in a manner that everyone is able to understand without having to seek clarification. Robert Mager in his book on preparing objectives indicates that a meaningfully stated outcome would be one that communicates to the staff the intent of the individual who stated it.[18] "The statement which communicates best will be one which describes the terminal behavior of the learner well enough to prevent misinterpretation."[19]

Time is another consideration when writing desired outcomes. The time limits should be precise for evaluation purposes but should not be so rigid that changes cannot readily be made based on reassessment of the priorities and necessary outcomes. It is important to remember to state the desired outcomes in terms of client behaviors rather than nurse behaviors, in keeping with the ANA *Standards of Nursing Practice.*[20] The *Standards* can be utilized as useful criteria for evaluating patient care.

The second stage in nursing care planning is the identification of nursing actions for each nursing diagnosis, based on carefully thought out scientific rationale. The nursing action tells what kind of nursing care is to be done to effectively meet the client's problem. Nursing actions should be precisely spelled out. These actions are part of the scheme for providing good nursing care. In planning for nursing care, it is important to include a statement of the desired changes in behavior that are to be brought about by the nursing actions. These desired outcomes are associated with goals and objectives.

Nursing actions can be said to be hypotheses established for testing if they contribute to the solution of the problem. It is up to the nurse in conjunction with the client and/or family to select appropriate actions that will produce the desired results. In selecting these nursing actions, it is important to analyze the options available and to determine the probability of success in reaching the objective. Sometimes compromises must be made in order to provide the best care for the client, and the nurse needs to be aware of this when writing nursing actions.

The nursing care plan deals with actual as well as potential problems. Nursing actions are based on scientific principles and theories of nursing and need to be specific. The plan serves as a means for resolving the problems and meeting established goals in an orderly fashion. Also, it provides a means for organization, giving direction and meaning to the nursing action used in helping the client and/or family to resolve his/her problem. A plan of action is essential in that it aids in the utilization of time efficiently, thus saving time and energy by providing essential data for those individuals responsible for giving care.

Since the client's condition is continuously changing, the written nursing care plan needs to reflect these changes. Therefore planning becomes a continuous process based on evaluation and reassessment and is the most efficient way of keeping all individuals involved in the client's care informed of modifications in the plan of nursing care.

Implementation

After planning, implementation is the next or fourth phase of the nursing process. Implementation refers to the action or actions initiated to accomplish defined goals and objectives.[21] Implementation is often considered as the actual giving of nursing care. It is putting the plan into action. Other terms used to describe this part of the process are *action* or *intervention*. According to *The Random House Dictionary*, the two words *implementation* and *intervention* are not synonymous.[22] The definition of implementation is "to put into effect according to or by means of a definite plan or procedures." Intervention is defined as "interposition or interference of one state in the affairs of another, a coming between." Therefore the term *implementation* seems more appropriate to describe this phase of the process if nursing actions are to follow from stated goals and objectives.

Since the nursing process is interpersonal in nature, it must take place between the nurse and the client. The client may be a person, a group, a family, or even a community. The beliefs that the nurse and the client have about human beings, nurses, clients, and interactions between nurses and clients will affect the types of actions that they both consider appropriate. If human beings are considered unique, then nursing actions should reflect this uniqueness. Therefore, the philosophy of nursing that a nurse develops will affect the nursing actions that he/she uses in meeting the needs of clients. Helen Yura and Mary Walsh in their book *The Nursing Process* indicate that the implementation phase of the nursing process draws heavily on the intellectual, interpersonal, and technical skills of the nurse.[23] Even though the focus is on action, the action is intellectual, interpersonal, and technical in nature.

The implementation phase begins when the nurse considers various alternative actions and selects those most suitable to achieve the planned goals and objectives. Just as goals and objectives have priorities in the plan, actions may also have priorities. Nursing actions may be carried out by the nurse who developed the nursing care plan or by other nurses or nursing assistants. Nursing actions may also be carried out by the client and/or family. To carry out a nursing action, the nurse refers back to the plan for additional information. Many nursing actions fall into the broad categories of counseling, teaching, providing physical care, carrying out delegated medical therapy, coordination of resources, referral to other sources of help, and therapeutic communication (verbal and nonverbal).

Based on the goals and objectives for Mrs. James, as discussed on page 18, there are several nursing actions that could be implemented. For example, under objective 1, the following actions could be considered:

1. Establish an agreed upon time when Mrs. James and her family could meet with the nurse in their home during the next week.
2. Establish baseline knowledge about Mrs. James's and the family members' understanding of basic food groups.
3. Bring chart and booklets containing information about the four basic food groups to Mrs. James's home.
4. Teach family about using the four basic food groups for good nutrition (base teaching on information gained from baseline knowledge).
5. Focus on the value of the food groups for each family member based on age, height, weight, and activity.
6. Request a return demonstration in which Mrs. James and other family members will identify foods by placing the food in a food group and will state why each food group is important.

For every nursing action, the client responds as a total person or as a whole. The concept of *holism*, which states that a person is more than the sum of that person's parts, means that the nurse may be treating a person's leg, but the person will respond as a whole person.[24] The concept is useful in thinking about the consequences of any nursing actions. For example, the simple action of turning the patient every two hours will have a variety of consequences. Some of these consequences should or could be: (1) increased circulation, (2) improved muscle tone, (3) improved breathing, (4) less flatus (gas) in the intestinal tract, (5) prevention of pressure sores, (6) increased or decreased pain, (7) opportunity for communication with care giver, (8) increased ability to socialize with patient in next bed, and (9) increased or decreased ability to reach articles at bedside. There may be other consequences that could not have been predicted, such as an opportunity to express values or beliefs. Therefore, in planning nursing actions, it is important to consider the cluster of consequences of both positive and negative value that could be expected to occur with and following each action.[25] Utilizing this knowledge will help the nurse in selecting the most appropriate actions. Even though not all consequences are predictable for a specific client, it is possible to develop a knowledge of expected consequences. Knowledge of consequences is an important aspect of the implementation phase of the nursing process. The implementation phase is completed when the nursing actions are finished and results are recorded.

Evaluation

Evaluation is the fifth and final phase of the nursing process. It may be defined as the appraisal of the client's behavioral changes due to the action of the nurse.[26] Although evaluation is considered to be the final phase, it frequently does not end the process. As we mentioned earlier in this chapter, evaluation may lead to reassessment, which in turn may result in the nursing process beginning all over again. The main questions to ask in evaluation are: Was the care effective? Were the goals and objectives met? Were there identifiable changes in the client/patient behavior? If so, why? If not, why not? Was I able to predict the expected consequences of nursing actions? These questions help the nurse to determine which problems have been solved and which problems need to be reassessed and replanned. Unsolved problems cannot be assumed to reflect faulty data collection or inadequate data collection; rather each part of the nursing process may need to be evaluated to determine the cause of ineffective actions.

The key to appropriately evaluating nurse/client actions lies in the planning phase of the process. If objectives are described in behavioral terms with the expected outcome clearly stated, then it is much easier to determine whether or not the nurse/client actions were successful. These objectives become the criteria for evaluating nurse/client actions. Just as goals should be mutually set with a client/patient, whenever possible, it is also important for the nurse and client to mutually establish the objectives (criteria for evaluation).

According to Dolores Little and Doris Carnevali,[27] evaluation consists of three sequential steps:

1. Selecting criteria (objectives) that will guide the nurse's observation to specified areas of the client's anticipated behavioral changes related to the diagnosis and goals.
2. Collecting specific evidence (data) after goals have been set and client-nurse activities have taken place.
3. Comparing the evidence collected to the criteria and baseline data (if available); then making judgments about the nature of the behavioral change (such as direction, stability, achievement).

Step 1 has been briefly discussed in relation to the planning phase of the process. In addition to stating the desired behavior change, it is also important for the nurse to decide how the change will be measured and when it will be measured.

Step 2 involves the collection of evidence (data). Although data are collected in both assessment and evaluation, the data collection during evaluation is utilized differently from data collected during assessment. In assessment, data are collected for the purpose of making a nursing diagnosis. In evaluation, data are collected as evidence to determine whether the goals and objectives were met. This is an important difference to note in using the nursing process.

Step 3 in evaluation is the one that often is the most difficult because it is easy to use different measurements in making judgments. For example, if a nurse observed that a client "ate well," would this mean the same thing to the client or to another nurse? "Ate well" could be interpreted to mean that the client was able to chew, swallow, and digest the food with no difficulty, or it could refer to the amount and kind of food consumed. Therefore, in evaluation it is not only important to determine the criteria (objectives) but also to determine the exact way(s) in which evidence will be gathered and interpreted to ascertain whether the criteria were met.

In the third step, baseline data refer to information that should be collected in the assessment of the client. To observe a change and to measure a change, the nurse must know the current status of the client or the base from which the change will take place. An example of baseline data could be the weight of the client on initial contact.

In the situation regarding Mrs. James, objectives were mutually set in measurable terms. Using Little and Carnevali's Step 1, it is possible to select criteria for measuring the first objective (identify the basic four food groups from a chart). The criteria set may include eighteen out of twenty foods correctly identified. If at the end of Week I, Mrs. James could identify nineteen foods correctly by food groups, then objective 1 would be evaluated as "accomplished." Specific evidence has been collected (Step 2) and compared to the criteria (Step 3). Baseline data were also obtained so that change in knowledge about food groups could be measured.

Under objective 2 (prepare a shopping list to include at least two foods from each group by the end of Week I), the criteria established could be:

1. The shopping list will include all foods essential for preparing three meals per day for seven days.
2. Two foods from each food group would be included on the shopping list.

In looking at the shopping list, the nurse discovered that no red meats were included, therefore creating a limited use of one food group. Mrs. James revealed that her husband did not believe in eating these animals. This information would be included as reassessment data, and the nurse would have to collect more information to help Mrs. James in meeting this objective.

When objectives have not been met, reassessment should occur and the process will begin again. If the evaluation shows that the nurse/client objectives have been met, the nursing process is complete at that particular point in time.

SUMMARY

In summary, the nursing process is the "tool" or methodology of professional nursing that helps nurses arrive at decisions and helps them predict and evaluate consequences. To use the nursing process successfully, a nurse needs to apply concepts and theories from nursing; from biological, physical, and behavioral sciences; and from the humanities, in order to provide a rationale for decision making, judgments, interpersonal relationships, and actions. The five components considered necessary to the nursing process are: assessment, nursing diagnosis, planning, implementation, and evaluation.

It is expected that students learning about the use of the nursing process will need to use many references and resources to augment their knowledge and skills as they proceed through their nursing program.

NOTES

1. Helen Yura and Mary B. Walsh, *The Nursing Process: Assessing, Planning, Implementing, Evaluating,* 2nd ed. (New York: Appleton-Century-Crofts, 1973), p. 69.
2. Fay Louise Bower, *The Process of Planning Nursing Care–A Model for Practice* (St. Louis, Mo.: The C. V. Mosby Co., 1977), p. 11.
3. Pamela Holsclaw Mitchell, *Concepts Basic to Nursing* (New York: McGraw-Hill Book Company, 1973), p. 71.
4. Ann Marriner, *The Nursing Process: A Scientific Approach to Nursing Care* (St. Louis, Mo.: The C. V. Mosby Co., 1975), p. 1.
5. Bower, *The Process of Planning,* pp. 10–11.
6. Judith Bloom Walter, Geraldine P. Pardee, and Doris M. Malbo, *Dynamics of Problem-Oriented Approaches: Patient Care and Documentation* (Philadelphia: J. B. Lippincott Co., 1976), pp. 32–39.
7. Bower, *The Process of Planning,* pp. 11–13, 48–70.
8. Donna S. Zimmerman and Carol Gohrke, "The Goal-Directed Nursing Approach: It Does Work," *The Nursing Process: A Scientific Approach,* Ann Marriner, compiler (St. Louis, Mo.: The C. V. Mosby Co., 1975), p. 150.
9. Lucille Lewis, *Planning Patient Care* (Dubuque, Iowa: Wm. C. Brown Publishers, 1976), Chapter 3.
10. Congress for Nursing Practice, *Standards of Nursing Practice* (Kansas City, Mo.: American Nurses' Association, 1973).
11. Elizabeth Anne Mahoney, Laurie Verdisco, and Lillie Shortridge, *How to Collect and Record a Health History* (Philadelphia: J. B. Lippincott Co., 1976), pp. 9–52.
12. Ibid., p. 5.
13. Dolores Little and Doris Carnevali, *Nursing Care Planning,* 2nd ed. (Philadelphia: J. B. Lippincott Co., 1976), p. 12.
14. Abraham Maslow, *Motivation and Personality* (New York: Harper and Row, Publishers, 1954).
15. E. H. Erikson, *Childhood and Society* (New York: W. W. Norton & Company, Inc., 1963), pp. 247–274.
16. *Self-Evaluation Report,* paper submitted to the National League for Nursing (Dayton, Ohio: Wright State University, School of Nursing, September, 1976), p. 96.
17. Ibid.
18. Robert Mager, *Preparing Instructional Objectives* (Palo Alto, Calif.: Fearon Publishers, Inc., 1962), p. 12.

19. Ibid., p. 11.
20. Congress for Nursing Practice, *Standards of Nursing Practice* (Kansas City, Mo., 1973).
21. *Self Evaluation Report*, p. 96.
22. *The Random House Dictionary of the English Language* (New York: Random House, Inc., 1966).
23. Yura and Walsh, *The Nursing Process*, p. 108.
24. Jan Christiaan Smuts, *Toward a Better World* (New York: World Book Company, distributed by Duell, Sloan and Pearce, 1944), pp. 123–133.
25. Marjorie L. Byrne and Lida F. Thompson, *Key Concepts for the Study and Practice of Nursing* (St. Louis, Mo.: The C. V. Mosby Co., 1972), pp. 67–75.
26. Ibid., Chapter 6.
27. Little and Carnevali, *Nursing Care Planning*, p. 230.

3

FLORENCE NIGHTINGALE

Gertrude Torres

Florence Nightingale (1820–1910) was born to English parents while they were on a trip to Florence, Italy. Her greatest achievement was the establishment of the concept of formal preparation for the practice of nursing; thus, the profession of nursing started with her commitment to the care of the sick.

Miss Nightingale's fame spread rapidly after she and a group of devoted women cared for the sick during the Crimean War. She was a proficient bedside nurse with a great concern for the soldiers. An account of her nightly rounds with her lamp ("The Lady with the Lamp") was given special attention by Henry Wadsworth Longfellow.

Organized nursing began in the mid-1800s with the leadership of Florence Nightingale. Before her era, nursing care was done by paupers and drunkards, persons unfit for any other type of work. Hospitals were places where the poor frequently suffered more from the environment than from the disease that brought them there. Surgery without anesthesia, little or no sanitation, and filth within hospitals were prevalent everywhere.

Nightingale's beliefs about nursing form the basic foundation on which nursing care is practiced today. Her religious convictions and military nursing experience during the Crimean War had a strong influence on her approach and beliefs about the care of the sick. Her writing ability, which is well demonstrated in her *Notes on Nursing*,[1] can be attributed to her education, which was achieved mainly through her father's tutoring. She traveled extensively and had the ability to deal in government and politics. Many have called her a genius. Thus, in understanding her theoretical approach to professional nursing, the reader needs to keep in mind her unique characteristics in relationship to the place of a woman of the mid-nineteenth century.

Nightingale did not specifically approach her writings in the context of today's terminology, that of concepts and theories. Yet these writings about nursing care can be interpreted to reflect the present emphasis on a theoretical approach to the nursing process. There may be the temptation to see her ideas as "old-fashioned" or "out-of-date." This must be avoided since many of her sound ideas about nursing are still not being universally carried out in contemporary practice.

NIGHTINGALE'S ENVIRONMENTAL THEORY OF NURSING

The core concept that is most reflective of Nightingale's writings is that of environment. Although she tends to emphasize the physical more than the psychological or social environment, this needs to be viewed in the context of her time and her activities as a nurse leader in a war-torn environment. It is understandable that she, having witnessed in the early 1850s the filth, vermin, and death within an enormous barracks hospital, would focus so heavily on improving the environment to assist soldiers to merely survive. Through such an emphasis, the death rate went from a staggering 42 per 100 to a low of 22 per 1000. This success gave her a strong data base on which to view nursing in her own unique way.

The environment is viewed as all the external conditions and influences affecting the life and development of an organism and capable of preventing, suppressing, or contributing to disease or death.[2] Nightingale's writing speaks of providing such things as ventilation, clean air and water, cleanliness, and warmth, so the reparative process that nature has instituted will not be hindered. Assisting patients toward the retention of their vital powers by meeting their needs is viewed as a goal of nursing. The flavor of her beliefs is expressed when she speaks of the environmental elements that disturb health, such as dirt, dampness, chills, drafts, smells, and darkness.[3]

Medical practice is not viewed as a curative process but as having the function of assisting nature. Thus, nursing is also a noncurative practice in which the patient is put in the best condition for nature to act. This condition was seen by her as enhanced by providing an environment conducive to health promotion.

At this point it is helpful to think of a patient who has had surgery, such as an appendectomy, and relate what Nightingale proposes. Medicine is seen as functioning to remove the diseased part, whereas nursing places the patient in an environment in which nature can assist postoperative patients to reach their optimum health condition. This approach to nursing is as valid today as it was over one hundred years ago, in spite of the fact that both in homes and in hospitals the environment today is more sophisticated in structure. This should be kept in mind as the theory is viewed in more detail. Much of Nightingale's theory is noted in her writing, *Notes on Nursing*.[4]

Table 3-1 demonstrates her major areas of environmental concentration: ventilation, warmth, effluvia, noise, and light. Keep in mind that it is the interrelationship of this concept of a healthy environment with the practice of nursing, as seen by Florence Nightingale, that offers us a basic theory of nursing practice.

Ventilation, especially with increased fresh air, provided without drafts, is of primary importance. *Light* refers to sunlight for the most part, and is secondary. *Warmth, noise,* and *effluvia* (smells) are seen as areas in which attention must be given in order to provide a positive environment.

In utilizing this basic concept—the environment—within the nursing process, it becomes evident that the practitioner must view the patient in a particular context. For example, review the following situation:

Situation 1. Mrs. Anderson, a public health nurse, has just visited Mrs. Rose, an eighty-year-old arthritic patient who lives alone in a small rural community. Since Mrs. Rose has difficulty ambulating, her neighbors visit her often to assist her in any way they can. One of these neighbors requested that Mrs. Anderson visit to assess the situation.

On entering Mrs. Rose's home, Mrs. Anderson was made aware of the lack of fresh air, the darkness in the environment caused by old dusty drapes covering the windows, and a draft in the bedroom. Mrs.

Table 3-1

Nightingale's Environmental Concepts

Major Areas of Concentration	Examples
Ventilation	Fresh air, which is of primary importance, can be achieved through open windows. Corrupt, stagnant, and musty air breeds disease. An outlet is needed for impure air. Drafts caused by open windows and doors are to be avoided. Dirty carpets and furniture are a source of impurity in the air.
Warmth	Guarding against the loss of vital heat is essential to the patient's recovery. Chilling is to be avoided. Hot bottles, bricks, and drinks should be used to restore lost heat.
Effluvia (smells)	Sewer air is to be avoided, and care is needed to get rid of noxious body odor caused by disease. Chamber utensils should be odor-free and out of sight. Fumigations and disinfectants should not be used but the offensive substance removed.
Noise	Intermittent sudden noise causes greater excitement than continuous noise, especially during the patient's first sleep. The more the patient sleeps peacefully, the greater his ability to sleep will be. Walking lightly, whispering, or discussing a patient's condition just outside his room is cruel.
Light	Second only to the need for fresh air is the value of light. Beds should be placed in such a position as to allow the patient to see out the window—the sky and sunlight.

Rose was found sitting in an old chair that provided little or no view of the world around her.

After her visit, Mrs. Anderson contacted Mrs. Rose's neighbors to set up a plan to improve her environment. The drapes were to be removed and replaced by simple curtains that would let the morning sun enter the home. The windows were to be opened in keeping with the weather during specific periods of the day, with care given to reduce drafts. Mrs. Rose's favorite chair was to be placed in such a way that she could look out the window to watch the neighbors coming and going.

This example is not to be viewed as offering a complete assessment of Mrs. Rose, but to point out how Nightingale's basic environmental concept, interrelated with the nursing process, can give us specific directions.

To Nightingale the environment of the patient was quite encompassing. Although she did not specifically distinguish among the physical, social, or psychological environments as such, she speaks of all three in the practice of nursing.

Admittedly, emphasis is placed on the physical environment of the patient. In the context of her time this was essential if lives were to be saved and nursing was to take its proper place as a profession. It is when an optimum physical environment exists that greater attention can be given to the emotional needs of the patient as well as to the prevention of disease.

Figure 3-1 offers a view of the theory created by Nightingale. The key point is diagrammed in the center of the triangle—patient condition and nature. Here the thrust of environment is on the patient and nature functioning together to allow the reparative process to occur. The three components—physical, social, and psychological—need to be viewed as interrelating rather than as separate distinct parts. The cleanliness of the physical environment has a direct bearing on the prevention of disease and mortality rates within the social environment

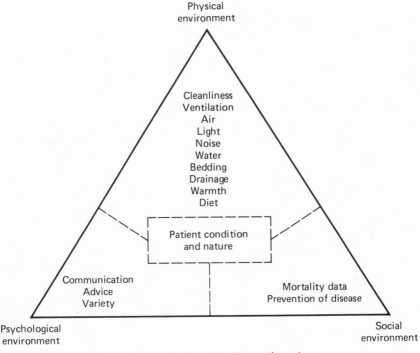

Figure 3-1. Nightingale's theory of nursing.

of the community. (Also, all patients' psychological environments are strongly affected by physical surroundings.)

Physical Environment

As noted in Table 3-1, the basic environmental components are physical in nature and relate to such things as ventilation and warmth. These basic factors affect one's approach to all other aspects of the environment. Cleanliness is an encompassing notion related to all aspects of the physical environment in which the patient is found. The walls and entire room should not be dusty, smoky, or have a close odor.

A patient's bed must be clean, aired, warm, dry, and free from odor. One should provide an environment in which the patient can be easily cared for by others or self. The width, height, and placement of the bed should facilitate the activities of the patient. The bed should be placed in the best lighted spot, away from sudden noises and the odor of drainage. The position of the patient on the bed should be viewed in the context of supporting ventilation.

Psychological Environment

The effect of the mind on the body was fairly well accepted in Nightingale's time. However, there was a lack of understanding of exactly how the condition of the body as affected by the environment could affect the mind. Nightingale did recognize that a negative environment could cause physical stress, thereby affecting the patient's emotional climate. Therefore emphasis is placed on offering the patient a variety of activities to keep his mind stimulated. The view of the sunlight, the attractiveness of the food, and the offering of manual activities that stimulate the need to labor are all factors that assist the patient to survive emotionally. Boredom is viewed as painful.

Communication with the patient is viewed in the context of the total environment. Communication should not be hurried or allow for interruptions. When speaking with patients, it is important to sit down in front of them, unless other activities such as eating are occurring. The place one communicates with the physician and family about the patient is in the context of the environment of the patient. Outside the patients' rooms or within their hearing distance is viewed as inappropriate.

One should not encourage the sick by false hopes and advice about their illness. Rather, the emphasis here is on communicating about the world around them that they miss, or about good news that visitors can share. Again, patients are viewed in the context of the total environment.

Social Environment

Observation of the social environment, especially as related to specific data collections relating to illness, is essential to preventing disease. Thus, each nurse must use observational powers in dealing with specific cases rather than be comfortable with data addressing the "average" patient.

Closely related to the community-social environment are those notions already discussed in relation to the individual patient—that is, physical environment such as clean air, water, and proper drainage or sewage. The patient's *total* environment not only includes the patient's home or hospital room but the total community influencing that specific environment.

NIGHTINGALE'S THEORY OF NURSING AS RELATED TO SCIENTIFIC THEORIES

Nightingale's theory of nursing is closely related to scientific theories frequently used in nursing practice today. Most significant are the theories of adaptation, need, and stress.

Adaptation

Adaptation reflects man's adjustments to forces that confront him. Such forces are viewed in the context of the total environment in which man finds himself. The success or nonsuccess of the adaptive responses of man can be seen by reviewing the environmental forces described by Nightingale. Man's ability to allow nature to act on his behalf as influenced by his environment will lead to adaptive or maladaptive responses. A patient who finds himself in a cold, dusty, poorly ventilated environment will have to use much of his available energy for adapting to his environment rather than for recovering from his illness.

To put this in the context of the present, one should note that during the Vietnam War injured soldiers were quickly airlifted to casualty stations in which they were treated before being sent to nearby hospitals for more complete care. In comparison to previous treatment of the injured, this led to a much lower death rate. Admittedly, this closely relates to improved medical care, but it should also be noted that removing the injured from a poor environment as soon as possible allowed nature to act on the patient's behalf—the Nightingale theory.

Need Theory

Need theories, especially Maslow's,[5] basically recognize theories given emphasis by Nightingale: for example, the need for oxygenation viewed in the context of fresh air, ventilation, and the need for a safe environment as related to proper drainage and clean water. Need theories stress man's ability to survive in the context of how well these needs are met. An environment that strongly supports man's basic physiological needs is essential. Maslow's emphasis on an hierarchical order of needs places physiological needs as primary, whereas emotional and social needs have less significance for survival.[6] Again, Nightingale's emphasis on the physical environment that affects the physiological functioning of man supports Maslow's theory.

Need theories frequently emphasize providing novelty and activities and encouraging exploration of the environment. Nightingale advised against having the patient suffer boredom from staring at four blank walls all day long. Today the literature speaks of sensory deprivation—demonstrated by boredom, daydreaming, and a lack of concentration.

Stress Theory

Stress involves a threat or a change in the environment in which an individual must cope. Stress can be positive or negative depending on its end result. Stress can encourage a person to take positive action toward a desired goal or need, or it can cause exhaustion if the stress is so intense that the individual is unable to cope. Nightingale emphasized placing the patient in an optimum environment so that there would be a minimum of outside stressors. For example, slow quiet movements, whispering, or sudden noises were viewed as causing stress, whereas purposeful quick actions were seen as more appropriate.

However, suddenly waking the patient causes great excitement and can be viewed as a negative stressor.

The number and duration of stressors have a strong influence on man's ability to cope. In reviewing the major components of Nightingale s theory, the greater the degree of poor air, poor water, poor light, and other negative environmental factors, and the longer the duration, the lesser the potential for the patient to cope with his illness. As a matter of fact, given a healthy individual within a poor environment with multiple stressors of long duration, illness would soon occur.

Situation II. Mrs. Kerr is a seventy-year-old resident who lives in an old local nursing home. She is rarely visited by her only living relative, a brother who is several years older. Several years ago she became partially immobile on her right side and continues to have difficulty walking around the home. When reminded, she is able to go to the dining room for meals but eats very little. Her environment consists of a two-bed room, which she shares with an eighty-year-old woman who is unaware of her surroundings. On admission, Mrs. Kerr was not able to bring any of her own belongings except for a few clothes. When communicating with her, she remembers the "old" days when she taught at the local elementary school. She seldom initiates a conversation and spends most of her time sitting in a chair in the lounge, apparently watching television.

The above situation is quite typical of a resident within today's nursing homes. In utilizing the nursing process with a focus on Nightingale's theory, it is essential to focus on Mrs. Kerr's environment and her reaction to it, rather than specifically on her as a resident. Table 3-2 reflects the use of the Nightingale theory.

The major emphasis in this situation is to restructure the immediate environment around Mrs. Kerr so that nature can act to maintain her optimum condition. With additional reassessment and evaluation, much can be done to prolong a healthy life and promote total comfort. It is possible, after such assessment, that the environment of the nursing home may be destructive to Mrs. Kerr's health. Alternatives may need to be sought. By the application of adaptation, need, and stress theories to this situation, in terms of the environment, the base for the practice of nursing becomes more theoretically sound.

Some of the questions that might be used to guide the practitioner in implementing Nightingale's theory in situations like Mrs. Kerr's are:

1. Is the environment the most crucial factor in the effective care of Mrs. Kerr?
2. What adaptations can be made within such environments that will facilitate optimum nursing care?
3. Do adjustments within the environment lead patients to a more optimum state of health and prolong their life?
4. Does the amount of stress within such environments affect both the residents and the nurse?

Table 3-2

Nightingale's Theory Applied to the Nursing Process

Nursing Process Phases	Mrs. Kerr
Assessment— Data available	Seventy-year-old woman who has partial paralysis of her right side. Can move about the environment. The home offers some alternatives to the resident's surroundings—a dining room, bedroom, and television lounge. Visitors from the outside are allowed. Residents are not encouraged to bring meaningful things with them to the home. The only sensory stimulation is one television set. During periods of eating, food intake is poor.
Data not provided	Inadequate information on the following: adequacy of ventilation, presence of drafts, sudden noises, cleanliness of surroundings, variety of dietary offerings, opportunities to communicate with others, variety of stimulus provided, specific physical limitations, previous nursing observation, odors present throughout the home, method of disposal of human wastes, amount of sunlight and artificial light.
Analysis of data	Basically, there is a lack of specific data, especially relating to the total environment of the nursing home. Thus, an analysis at this time must be viewed as tentative in nature until a reassessment can be done.
Nursing Diagnosis	Nonstimulating environment.
Goals	Increased communication. Provide for an optimum environment that will facilitate health.
Implementation	Increase stimulus through a greater exposure to sunlight and fresh air. Place Mrs. Kerr in a room that will increase the amount of interaction she has with others.
Evaluation	Observe effect of a changing environment on her health state.

5. What hierarchy of needs is met in such an environment?

As an approach to the practice of nursing, Nightingale's theory is as valid today as it was over one hundred years ago. Within the hospital environment, much can be done to reduce stress, improve adaptation, and meet patient needs through minor adjustments that can be made by the professional nurse. Some examples are the following: the placement of a patient's bed within the room to provide a view of the outside world or sunlight; the encouraging and educating of visitors to provide a greater amount of variety or stimulation within the environment; the less frequent, sudden awakening of patients; and the provision for a quiet, unhurried atmosphere. Although today's hospitals have clean air through the air conditioning system, and clean water through more sophisticated plumbing systems, they still have drafty, odorous environments created by the lack of attention to such details.

Much of Nightingale's theory might be viewed as involving basic common sense, such as giving attention to the cleanliness of a patient's surroundings, keeping chills away, and providing adequate lighting to read. Yet, such things are frequently taken for granted and are often forgotten.

SUMMARY

Nightingale's major focus was on the environment of the patient. Nursing was viewed as distinct from medicine and focused on providing an environment that allowed nature to act on behalf of the patient. Environmental factors involved clean air, water, control of noise, proper drainage, reduction of chills, and variety of activities. Nightingale emphasized fresh air as primary and good lighting as secondary to the effective care of the patient. Other theories most closely related to her writings are adaptation, need, and stress. In utilizing her theory within the nursing process, the focus is on how the environment affects the patient. Implementation involves adjustments to inadequate environments. Nightingale's theory is as appropriate today as a theoretical base for practice as it was during her time of practice in the mid-1800s. It is the foundation on which all other theories in nursing should be viewed.

NOTES

1. Florence Nightingale, *Notes on Nursing* (New York: Dover Publications, Inc., 1969).
2. Ruth Murray and Judith Zentner, *Nursing Concepts for Health Promotion* (Englewood Cliffs, N.J.: Prentice-Hall, Inc., 1975), p. 149.
3. Nightingale, *Notes on Nursing.*
4. Ibid.
5. Abraham Maslow, *Motivation and Personality* (New York: Harper and Row, Publishers, 1954).
6. Ibid.

REFERENCES

AULD, MARGARET E., and LINDA HULTHEN BIRUM, *The Challenge of Nursing: A Book of Readings.* St. Louis, Mo.: The C. V. Mosby Co., 1973.

BYRNE, MARJORIE L., and LIDA F. THOMPSON, *Key Concepts for the Study and Practice of Nursing.* St. Louis, Mo.: The C. V. Mosby Co., 1972.

MURRAY, RUTH, and JUDITH ZENTNER, *Nursing Concepts for Health Promotion.* Englewood Cliffs, N.J.: Prentice-Hall, Inc., 1975.

NIGHTINGALE, FLORENCE, *Notes on Nursing.* New York: Dover Publications, Inc., 1969.

4

LYDIA E. HALL

Kathleen Hale and Julia B. George

Lydia E. Hall received her basic nursing education at York Hospital School of Nursing in York, Pennsylvania. Both her B.S. and M.A. are from Teacher's College, Columbia University, New York.

Lydia Hall was the first director of the Loeb Center for Nursing and Rehabilitation. Her experience in nursing spans the clinical, educational, and supervisory components. Her publications include several articles on the definition of nursing and quality of care. Lydia Hall has put forth what she considers a basic philosophy of nursing, upon which the nurse may base patient care. This philosophy is used as a working reality at the Loeb Center for Nursing.

LOEB CENTER FOR NURSING AND REHABILITATION

Lydia Hall originated the philosophy of care of Loeb Center at Montefiore Hospital, Bronx, New York. Loeb Center opened in January 1963 to provide professional nursing care to persons who are past the acute stage of illness. The center's functioning concept is that the need for professional nursing care increases as the need for medical care decreases.

Those in need of continued professional care who are sixteen years of age or older and are no longer experiencing an acute biological disturbance are transferred from the acute care hospital to Loeb Center. Good candidates for care at Loeb are those who have a desire to come to Loeb, are recommended by their physicians, and possess a favorable potential for recovery and return to the community.

Physically, Loeb Center has a capacity of eighty beds and is attached to Montefiore Hospital. The rooms are arranged with patient comfort and maneuverability as first priority. The patients also have access to a large communal dining room. The primary care givers are registered professional nurses with nonpatient care activities being supplied by messenger-attendants and secretaries.

> Loeb's primary purpose was and is to demonstrate that high quality nursing care given by registered nurses, in a non-directive setting, offers a supportive service to people in the post-acute phase of their illness that enables them to recover sooner, and to leave the center able to cope with themselves and what they must face in the future.[1]

To create a nondirective setting, there are very few rules, no routines, no schedules, and no dictated mealtimes or specified visiting hours.[2] The nurses at Loeb strive to help the patient determine and clarify goals and, with the patient, work out ways to achieve the goal at the individual's pace, consistent with the medical treatment plan and congruent with the patient's sense of self.[3]

LYDIA HALL'S THEORY OF NURSING

Lydia Hall presents her theory of nursing visually by drawing three interlocking circles, each circle presenting a particular aspect of nursing. The circles represent *care, core,* and *cure.*

The Care Circle

The care circle (Figure 4-1) represents the nurturing component of nursing and is exclusive to nursing. Involved in nurturing is the utilization of the factors that make up the concept of mothering (care and comfort of the person).

The professional nurse cares for the patient and helps complete

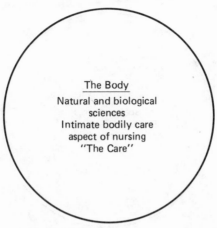

The Body
Natural and biological
sciences
Intimate bodily care
aspect of nursing
"The Care"

Figure 4-1. The care circle of patient care. (*From* Lydia Hall, *Nursing—What Is It?,* publication of the Virginia State Nurses' Association, Winter 1959, p. 1. Used with permission.)

such basic daily biological functions as eating, bathing, and dressing. Providing care for a patient at the basic needs level presents the nurse and patient with an opportunity for closeness. When this opportunity is developed to the fullest, the patient is given an opportunity to share and explore feelings with the nurse. When providing this care, the nurse has as a main goal the comfort of the patient.

When functioning in the care circle, the nurse applies knowledge of the natural and biological sciences to provide a strong theoretical base for nursing implementations. In interactions with the patient the nurse's role must be clearly defined. A strong theory base allows the nurse to incorporate closeness and nurturance while maintaining a professional status rather than a mothering status. The patient views the nurse as a potential comforter, one who provides care and comfort through the laying on of hands.

The Core Circle

The core circle (Figure 4-2) of patient care involves the therapeutic use of self and is shared with other members of the health team. The professional nurse, by developing an interpersonal relationship with the patient (as shown in the care circle, Figure 4-1), is able to help the patient verbally express feelings regarding the disease process. Through such expression the patient is able to gain self-identity and further develop toward maturity.

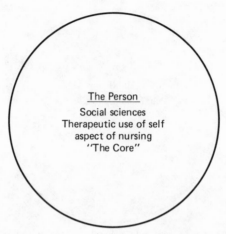

Figure 4-2. The core circle of patient care. (*From* Lydia Hall, *Nursing—What Is It?*, p. 1. Used with permission.)

The professional nurse, by use of the reflective technique (acting as a mirror for the patient), helps the patient look at and explore feelings regarding his or her current health status and related potential changes in life style. The nurse uses a freely offered closeness to help the patient bring into awareness the verbal and nonverbal messages being sent to others. Motivations are discovered through the process of bringing into awareness the feelings being experienced. The patient is now able to make conscious decisions based on understood and accepted feelings and motivations. The motivation and energy necessary for healing exist within the patient rather than in the health care team.

> To look at and listen to self is often too difficult without the help of a significant figure (nurturer) who has learned how to hold up a mirror and sounding board to invite the behaver to look and listen to himself. If he accepts the invitation, he will explore the concerns in his acts and as he listens to his exploration through the reflections of the nurse, he may uncover in sequence his difficulties, the problem area, his problem and eventually the threat which is dictating his out-of-control behavior.[4]

The Cure Circle

The cure circle of patient care (Figure 4-3) is shared with other members of the health team. The professional nurse helps the patient and family through the medical, surgical, and/or rehabilitative pre-

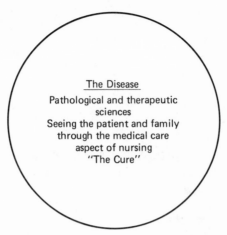

Figure 4-3. The cure circle of patient care. (*From* Lydia Hall, *Nursing—What Is It?*, p. 1. Used with permission.)

scriptions made by the physician. During this aspect of nursing care the nurse is an active advocate of the patient.

The nurse's role during the cure aspect is different from the care circle since many of the nurse's actions take on a negative quality of avoidance of pain rather than a positive quality of comforting. This is negative in the sense that the patient views the nurse as a potential cause of pain, involved in such actions as administering injections, versus the potential comforter who provided care and comfort.

Interaction of the Three Aspects of Nursing

The three aspects of nursing as Hall identifies them (Figure 4-4) do not function independently, but are interrelated, and they interact and change size depending on the patient's total course of progress. In the philosophy of Loeb Center the professional nurse functions most therapeutically when patients have entered this second stage of their hospital stay (i.e., where they are recuperating and are past the first acute stage).

During this stage, the care and core aspects are the most prominent, and the cure aspect is less prominent (see Figure 4-5). The size of the circles represents the degree to which the patient is progressing in each of the three areas. The professional nurse at this time is able to help the patient reach the core of his problem through the closeness provided by the care aspect of nursing.

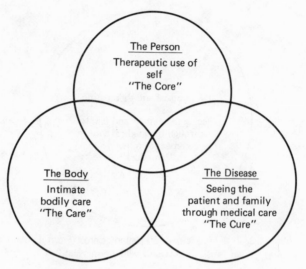

Figure 4-4. Hall's three aspects of nursing.

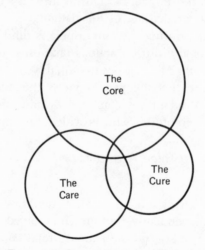

Figure 4-5. Care and core predominate.

HALL'S THEORY AND THE NURSING PROCESS

Hall places the motivation and energy needed for healing within the patient. This aspect of her theory influences the nurse's total approach to the five phases of the nursing process: assessment, diagnosis, planning, implementation, and evaluation.

The *assessment* phase involves collection of data about the health status of the individual. According to Hall, the process of data collection is directed for the benefit of the patient rather than for the benefit of the nurse. Data collection should be directed toward increasing the patient's self-awareness. Through use of observation and reflection, the nurse is able to assist the patient in becoming aware of both verbal and nonverbal behaviors. In the individual, increased awareness of feelings and needs in relation to health status increases his ability for self-healing.

The assessment phase also pertains to guiding the patient through the cure aspect of nursing. The health team collects biological data (physical and laboratory) to help the patient and family understand and progress through the medical regime.

The second phase is the *nursing diagnosis,* or statement of the patient's need or problem area. How a nurse envisions the nursing role will influence the interpretation of assessment data and conclusions reached. Viewing the patient as the power for self-healing will direct conclusions differently than if the healing power rests in the physician or nurse. The patient will be the one in control.

Planning involves setting priorities and mutually establishing patient-centered goals. The patient will decide what is of highest priority and also what goals are desirable.

The core is involved in planning. The role of the nurse is to use reflection to help the patient become aware of and understand needs, feelings, and motivations. Once motivations are clarified, Hall indicates the patient is the best person to set goals and arrange priorities. The nurse seeks to increase patient awareness and to support decision making based on the patient's new level of awareness. The nurse works with the patient to help keep the goals consistent with the medical prescription. The nurse needs to draw on a knowledge base in the social and scientific areas to present the patient with creative alternatives from which to choose.

Implementation involves the actual institution of the plan of care. This phase is the actual giving of nursing care. In the care circle intimate bodily care is given to the patient by the nurse. The nurse works *with* the patient, helping with bathing, dressing, eating, and other care and comfort needs.

The nurse also helps the patient and family through the cure aspect of nursing. She works with the patient and family to help them understand and implement the medical plan.

The professional nurse uses a "permissive non-directive teaching-learning approach" to implement nursing care, thus helping the patient reach the established goals.[5] This includes "helping the patient with his feelings, providing requested information and supporting patient-made decisions."[6]

Evaluation is the process of assessing the patient's progress toward the health goals. The evaluation phase of the process is directed toward deciding whether or not the patient is successful in reaching the established goals. The following questions would apply to the use of Hall's theory in the evaluation phase.

1. Is the patient learning "who he is, where he wants to go, and how he wants to get there?"[7]
2. Is the patient learning to understand and explore the feelings that underlie behavior?
3. Is the nurse helping the patient see motivations more clearly?
4. Are the patient's goals congruent with the medical regime? Is the patient successful in meeting the goals?
5. Is the patient physically more comfortable?

Whether or not a person is growing in self-awareness regarding his feelings and motivations can be recognized through changes in his outward behavior.

APPLICATION AND LIMITATIONS OF THE THEORY

In reviewing Hall's theory of nursing there are several areas that limit its application to patient care.

The first of these areas is the stage of illness. Hall applies her ideas of nursing to a patient who has passed the acute stage of biological stress; i.e., the patient who is experiencing the acute phase of illness is not included in Hall's approach to nursing care. However, it is possible to apply the care, core, and cure ideas to the care of those who are acutely ill. The acutely ill individual often needs care in relation to basic needs; he also needs core awareness of what is going on, and cure understanding of the plan of medical care.

A second limiting factor is age. Hall refers only to adult patients in the second stage of their illness. This eliminates all younger patients. Based on this theory Loeb Center admits only patients sixteen years of age and older.

A third limiting factor is the description of how to help a person toward self-awareness. The only tool of therapeutic communication discussed is reflection. By inference, all other techniques of therapeutic communication are eliminated. But reflection is not always the most effective technique to be used.

Fourth, the family is mentioned only in the cure circle. This means the nursing contact with families is used only in regard to the patient's own medical care. It does not allow for helping a family increase awareness of the family's self.

Finally, Hall's theory relates only to those who are ill. This would indicate no nursing contact with healthy individuals, families, or communities and negates the concept of health maintenance and preventive health care.

Basically, Hall's theory can be readily applied within the confines of the definition of adults past the acute stage of illness. However, this is too confining for a total view of nursing, which includes working with individuals, families, and communities throughout the life cycle and along a health continuum.

SUMMARY

Although Lydia Hall first presented her theory of nursing during the late 1950s and early 1960s, Loeb Center for Nursing and Rehabilitation is still using Hall's theory in providing patient care today.

Hall's theory of nursing involves three interlocking circles, each representing one aspect of nursing. The care aspect represents intimate bodily care of the patient. The core aspect deals with the innermost feelings and motivations of the patient. The cure aspect tells how the nurse helps the patient and family through the medical aspect of care. The main tool the nurse uses to help the patient realize his motivations and to grow in self-awareness is that of reflection.

Lydia Hall's theory may be used in the nursing process. The core, care, and cure aspects are applicable to each phase of the nursing process. The limitations of Hall's theory—illness orientation, age and family contact restrictions, use of reflection only—can be overcome by taking a broader view of care, core, and cure and by emphasizing the aspect that is most appropriate for a particular situation.

NOTES

1. Susan Bowar-Ferres, "Loeb Center and Its Philosophy of Nursing," *The American Journal of Nursing,* 75, no. 5 (May 1975), 810.
2. Ibid., p. 814.
3. Ibid., p. 813.
4. Lydia Hall, "Another View of Nursing Care and Quality," address given at Catholic University Workshop, Washington, D.C., 1965.
5. Bowar-Ferres, "Loeb Center and Its Philosophy of Nursing," p. 813.
6. Ibid.
7. Ibid.

REFERENCES

ALFANO, GENROSE, "Administration Means Working with Nurses," *The American Journal of Nursing,* vol. 64, no. 6 (June 1964).

BERNARDIN, ESTELLE, "Loeb Center—As the Staff Nurse Sees It," *The American Journal of Nursing,* vol. 64, no. 6 (June 1964).

BOWAR-FERRES, SUSAN, "Loeb Center and Its Philosophy of Nursing," *The American Journal of Nursing,* vol. 75, no. 5 (May 1975).

HALL, LYDIA, "Quality of Nursing Care," *Public Health News,* New Jersey State Department of Health, June 1955.

———, *Nursing—What Is It?* publication of the Virginia State Nurses Assn., Winter 1959.

———, "A Center for Nursing," *Nursing Outlook,* vol. II, no. 1 (November 1963).

———, "Another View of Nursing Care and Quality," address by L. E. Hall at Catholic University Workshop, Washington, D.C., 1965.

———, "The Loeb Center for Nursing and Rehabilitation at Montefiore Hospital and Medical Center," *International Journal of Nursing Studies,* vol. 6 (1969).

———, "Can Nursing Care Hasten Recovery?" *The American Journal of Nursing,* vol. 64, no. 6 (June 1964).

ISLER, CHARLOTTE, "New Concepts in Nursing Therapy, More Care as the Patient Improves," *R.N.* (June 1964).

5

VIRGINIA HENDERSON

Chiyoko Yamamoto Furukawa and Joan K. Howe

Virginia Henderson was born in Kansas City, Missouri, in 1897, the fifth child of a family of eight children. Most of her formative years were spent in Virginia, for her father practiced law in Washington, D.C.

Henderson's interest in nursing evolved during World War I from her desire to help the sick as well as the injured military personnel. She entered the Army School of Nursing in Washington and graduated from this school in 1921.

In 1926 Henderson attended Teachers College, Columbia University, and received a B.S. and M.A. degrees in nursing education. She taught at Teachers College from 1930 to 1948, emphasizing clinical practice using the analytical process.

Henderson is a recipient of numerous recognitions for her outstanding contributions to nursing. Her publications The Nature of Nursing *and* ICN Basic Principles of Nursing Care *are widely known and are translated into several foreign languages for the benefit of non-English-speaking nurses.* [1]

What is the practice of nursing? What specific functions do nurses perform? What are nursing's unique activities? Henderson created her definition of nursing in order to communicate her thoughts on these questions. She believed an occupation that provides service affecting human life must outline its functions, particularly if it is to be regarded as a profession.[2] Her formulation of the definition of nursing was influenced by her educational preparation and practice, by students and colleagues at Columbia University School of Nursing, and by other past and present nursing leaders. All these factors contributed to her thinking and helped delineate her beliefs about the unique function of the nurse. However, the major dominating force appears to be her own educational experiences and nursing practice, which gave her much insight into what nursing should be and how it should be focused. A description of Henderson's educational preparation and practice furnishes the basis on which to examine her definition of nursing.

EDUCATIONAL BACKGROUND AND PRACTICE

Henderson acknowledges her interpretation of the nurse's function as the synthesis of many influences, both positive and negative.[3] One major influence was her basic educational preparation in a general hospital, primarily at the Army School of Nursing in Washington. The emphasis of education there was on learning by doing, speed of performance, and technical competence. One's ability was measured against successful mastery of procedures such as catheterizations. The impersonal approach to care was used and was viewed as professional behavior. The importance of ethics was stressed as an assurance to compassion for humanity.[4]

Physician lectures to nursing students were a simplified version of instruction given to medical students. The emphasis on disease, diagnosis, and treatment regimen was a cut-and-dried approach to learning. With the aid of Annie W. Goodrich, dean of her school, Henderson recognized her own discontent with the regimentalized mode of patient care. She concluded this concept of nursing was simply an extension of medicine. At this stage of her education, Henderson yearned to see her teachers practice because the opportunity to observe a graduate nurse in practice was limited. This was an era when students were used to staff the hospital in return for their educational experience. From these thoughts it can be concluded that she lacked a role model. Clinical practice was viewed as self-learned while caring for the sick and wounded soldiers. The atmosphere was one of indebtedness to the patient for having served the country on the battlefields. Henderson describes the scene of nurse-patient relationship as a warm and generous one.[5] The nurse felt the need to do all she could, while the soldiers asked for little. This experience was viewed as unique, because in a civilian hospital there is a lack of the atmosphere of indebtedness to the patient for having served on the country's battlefields.

According to Henderson, the psychiatric affiliation, as the part of her preparation for nursing where human relations skills could have been learned, failed to materialize. Here again, the approach to patient care was on disease entities and treatment. The lack of understanding regarding the nurse's role in the prevention of mental illness or the cure of the psychiatric patient distressed Henderson. The experience left her with a sense of failure as a nurse. The only value of the psychiatric affiliation was the opportunity to gain some appreciation of mental illness.[6]

The pediatric nursing experience at the Boston Floating Hospital was more positive and introduced the concepts of patient-centered care, continuity of care, and tender loving care. The task-oriented approach could be discarded in this setting along with the regimented approach to care. However, there were other shortcomings identified in this setting. For example, the concept of family-centered care was lacking.[7] Parents were not allowed to visit their sick child, thus isolating the child just when parental supports were needed most. Also, there was no consideration given to knowledge about the home environment to better understand the needs of the child and the family.

Henderson's final experience as a student allowed her to view the community approach to nursing care at the Henry Street Visiting Nurse Agency in New York. In this setting, the formal approach to patient care that she had learned in a hospital was replaced. At Henry Street, she saw that the institutional type of regimen that is selected in a hospital did not consider the life style of the sick. Henderson noted that upon discharge the patient returned to the same environment that had originally led him or her to hospitalization.[8] Thus, she developed her skepticism of the care program given in a hospital. This kind of care only served as a stop-gap measure, without getting to the cause of the problem. The care given failed to consider the patient living outside the institution where behavioral controls were not available.

As a graduate nurse, Henderson worked for several years at the

Instructive Visiting Nurse Agency in Washington because she refused to accept the hospital system of nursing. She found this new experience rewarding and had the opportunity to institute her ideas about nursing.

The next position, which she held for five years, was teaching nursing students in a diploma program at the Norfolk Protestant Hospital in Virginia. She accepted this responsibility without further educational preparation because the institution needed her. This situation was not unique because many diploma schools had no teacher requirements. It was during this time that she recognized a need for more knowledge and clarification of the nursing functions. Thus she enrolled at Columbia Teachers College to learn the sciences and humanities relevant to nursing. It was during this time that the inquiry and analytic approach to nursing became important to her.

Following graduation, Henderson accepted the position of a teaching supervisor in the clinics of Strong Memorial Hospital in Rochester, New York, for a brief time. Subsequently, she taught at Columbia for twenty years, ending her teaching career in 1948. While at Columbia many of Henderson's ideas on nursing were implemented in the teaching of medical-surgical nursing; included were the patient-centered approach, the use of the nursing problem approach replacing the medical diagnoses model, emphasis on the field experiences for students, family follow-up care, and chronic illness care. She also established nursing clinics and encouraged coordination of care with other health professionals.

THE NEED FOR A DEFINITION
OF NURSING

There were two major reasons for the development of the definition of nursing by Henderson. First was her involvement with the revision of a nursing textbook, and second was her concern for licensure of nurses, as many states did not have this provision.

In preparing the 1939 revision of the *Textbook of the Principles and Practice of Nursing*, which she co-authored with the Canadian nurse Bertha Harmer, Henderson recognized the need to be clear about the functions of the nurse.[9] Henderson felt a textbook of nursing that serves as a main source in learning the practice of nursing should present a sound and definitive description of nursing. Furthermore, the principles and practice of nursing must be built upon and derived from the definition of the profession.

Her interest in defining nursing coincided with the question of licensure of the practitioner. The process of regulating nursing practice through licensure requires a definition of nursing to be explicitly stated in the Nurse Practice Acts. These acts provide the legal parameters for the nurse's functions in the care of consumers. The primary purpose of this legislative process is the protection of the public from unprepared practitioners as well as a method of providing a degree of control on the quality of nursing care delivered to the consumers.

Although official statements on the nursing function were available from the American Nurses' Association (ANA) in 1932 and 1937, Henderson viewed these statements as nonspecific and felt that they did not satisfy the question of what is nursing practice.[10] The 1955 ANA statement was improved by the incorporation of the independent function,* but Henderson still felt the definition was very general and too vague. The 1955 ANA statement suggested the nurse could observe, care for, and counsel the patient and could supervise other health personnel without herself being supervised by the physician (see quotation below). However, Henderson did not concur with the 1955 ANA statement because it limited the nurse to giving medications and doing treatment prescribed by the physician, and prohibited the nurse from diagnosing, prescribing, or correcting nursing care problems. Thus she viewed the statement as another unclear definition of nursing.[11] The 1955 ANA definition of nursing practice read as follows:

> The practice of professional nursing means the performance for compensation of any act in the observation, care, and counsel of the ill, injured, or infirm, or in the maintenance of health or prevention of illness of others, or in the supervision and teaching of other personnel, or the administration of medications and treatments as prescribed by a licensed physician or dentist; requiring substantial specialized judgment and skill and based on knowledge and application of the principles of biological, physical, and social science. The foregoing shall not be deemed to include arts of diagnosis or prescription of therapeutic or corrective measures.[12]

This statement was approved by the American Nurses' Association, Board of Directors, September 22, 1955.

*Independent functions are those actions that are self-directed.

Henderson's definition evolved as a result of her extensive experiences as a student, teacher, practitioner, and author. She was a participant in conferences that investigated and debated the nurse's function. The results of these gatherings were documented, but the circulation was limited to the participants and to concerned nursing leaders of that time.

In 1955, Henderson's first definition (see second quote below) was published in the revision of Harmer's textbook. This statement on nursing conveys the essence of her definition of nursing as it is known today. Therefore, it is noteworthy to compare and examine the influence of Harmer's 1922 definition to that of Henderson's, as the contents are similar and a relationship exists.

Harmer's 1922 Definition

Nursing is rooted in the needs of humanity and is founded on the ideal of service. Its object is not only to cure the sick and heal the wounded but to bring health and ease, rest, and comfort to mind and body, to shelter, nourish and practice and to minister to all those who are helpless or handicapped, young, aged or immature. Its object is to prevent disease and to preserve health. Nursing is, therefore, linked with every other social agency which strives for the prevention of disease and the preservation of health. The nurse finds herself not only concerned with the care of the individual but the health of people. [13]

Henderson's First (1955) Definition

Nursing is primarily assisting the individual (sick or well) in the performance of those activities contributing to health, or its recovery (or a peaceful death) that he would perform unaided if he had the necessary strength, will or knowledge. It is likewise the unique contribution of nursing to help the individual to be independent of such assistance as soon as possible. [14]

Henderson's definition abbreviated and consolidated Harmer's notions about nursing. Harmer's definition focused on disease prevention and health preservation. The need for linkage with other social agencies to strive for preventive care and the concern with the health of the people were given less or no emphasis by Henderson; she focused more on the individual.

The aspects of "teaching the individual proper habits of living relating to food, rest, exercise, recreation, sleep, and all the conditions which insure health of body and mind and increased resistance to disease"[15] were incorporated into Henderson's fourteen components of basic nursing care, as listed below. These components consist of "helping the patient with the following activities or providing conditions under which he can perform them unaided:"[16]

1. Breathe normally.
2. Eat and drink adequately.
3. Eliminate body wastes.
4. Move and maintain desirable postures.
5. Sleep and rest.
6. Select suitable clothing—dress and undress.
7. Maintain body temperature within normal range by adjusting clothing and modifying the environment.
8. Keep the body clean and well-groomed and protect the integument.
9. Avoid dangers in the environment and avoid injuring others.
10. Communicate with others in expressing emotions, needs, fears, or opinions.
11. Worship according to one's faith.
12. Work in such a way that there is a sense of accomplishment.
13. Play or participate in various forms of recreation.
14. Learn, discover, or satisfy the curiosity that leads to normal development and health and use of the available health facilities.

These components must be considered as a part of the definition of nursing to appreciate the essence of Henderson's thoughts.

In 1966, Henderson outlined her ultimate statement of the definition of nursing in *The Nature of Nursing.* She viewed this statement as "the crystallization of my ideas."

> The unique function of the nurse is to assist the individual, sick or well, in the performance of those activities contributing to health or its recovery (or to peaceful death) that he could perform unaided if he had the necessary strength, will or knowledge. And to do this in such a way as to help him gain independence as rapidly as possible.[17]

Henderson's definition of nursing in itself fails to fully acknowledge the main ideas and views she expounded. To comprehend the breadth of her thoughts about nursing incorporated in the definition and the fourteen components of basic nursing care, it is necessary to study her booklet, *Basic Principles of Nursing Care* (published by the International Council of Nurses in Geneva, 1972). Henderson believed her two statements, the "definition of nursing" and the "fourteen components," together outline the functions the nurse can initiate and control. [18]

As to the role of the nurse in carrying out the therapeutic plans of the physician, the nurse is expected to be a member of the medical team and is viewed as a prime helper to the patient in assuring the physician's prescriptions are instituted; this function is believed to foster a therapeutic relationship with the patient. [19] The concept of the nurse cooperating with other health workers is chiefly for the benefit of the patient in order to help him recover from his illness or to support him in death. The ideal situation for a nurse is to function as a fully participating team member, but to avoid any interference with the performance of the nurse's unique function. Henderson envisioned the unique function of the nurse is to identify and serve as a substitute for what the patient lacks to make him "complete," "whole," or "independent" with respect to physical strength, will, or knowledge to reach good health. [20]

Henderson further cautions the nurse from undertaking tasks that detract from the professional role and stresses that priority must be on the nurse's unique function. On the other hand, Henderson admits to situations where the nurse may assume the role of other health workers or function as a cook or plumber in order to supply the patient's obvious needs. [21] Thus, this position likens the nurse's role to that of a mother responding to the needs of a child.

This all-embracing role of Henderson's nurse has caused dissension with respect to the more generally accepted concept of the function of the nurse and her essential qualifications that differ from those of other health professionals. This role identification dilemma still exists today.

THEORETICAL BASIS OF HENDERSON'S DEFINITION OF NURSING

Henderson wrote her definition of nursing before the era of focus on concepts and theories about nursing. The primary problem to address up to that time dealt with the identification of the specific functions the nurse performs rather than with the theoretical basis for nursing practice. However, in the analysis of Henderson's definition of nursing and her fourteen components of basic nursing care, some inferences in relation to concepts emerge. For example, the concept of empathy could be derived from the statement the nurse must get "inside the skin" of the patients to understand and be sensitive to their needs.[22]

Henderson conveyed her thoughts and ideas about the importance of the fourteen components through her publications. If concepts are viewed as a method of transporting abstract thoughts and are similar to a definition of ideas, Henderson's definition of nursing supported by her fourteen components could be viewed as a concept.

The major theoretical basis for Henderson's definition of nursing is the factor of fundamental human needs. According to Henderson, Dr. Edward Thorndike's work in psychology furnished some generalization in the psychosocial area.[23] His research on the fundamental needs of man, including how people spend money and time, contributed to the realization that "illness was more than a state of dis-ease and a threat to life."[24] Henderson was thinking about how a patient's shelter needs are met in the hospital while other needs such as the freedom of movement, choices about eating, and invasion of privacy are not considered in most instances by the hospital personnel. Whether the individual is sick or well, the nurse needs to be cognizant of the inescapable human desire for food, shelter, and clothing; for love and approval; and for a sense of usefulness and mutual dependence in social relationships.[25]

If one were to select a human need theory that supports Henderson's definition of nursing, Maslow's hierarchy of needs may be most appropriate.[26] This hierarchy includes: (1) physiological needs, (2) safety needs, (3) belonging and love needs, (4) need for social esteem, and (5) need for self-actualization. Maslow considered man's responses to his needs as an integrated behavioral unit by emphasizing the relationships between the various needs. He believed that man functions holistically and seeks gratification of the most critical need for survival first; then afterward he seeks to meet needs that are less critical. When a need is met, gratification is achieved temporarily rather than permanently; and thus man is moving from satisfaction to seeking to meet his changing needs again and again.[27]

In relating Henderson's components of nursing care to Maslow's theory, it is clear that much of her focus is on the physiological and safety needs, with less emphasis on the other areas of need. Of the fourteen components a majority of them relate to the physiological and safety needs. Maslow's psychosocial elements such as social esteem and self-actualization could be matched to Henderson's components that refer to communication of emotions, worship, work accomplishment, recreation, and learning to satisfy curiosity with respect to normal development, health, and use of health facilities.

The concept of culture as it affects human needs is considered by Henderson to be those needs learned from the family and other social groups. She excluded from these needs specifically religious faith and ethics, as these serve man as a fixed point or guide to conduct.[28] These needs are not viewed as a specific desire to uphold one's belief in God but rather to do one's best to live up to whatever one's faith demands. Cultural differences and motivation influence human needs to the extent that some needs are stronger, and other needs come and go as satisfaction is achieved. Although recognizing these differences, it is equally important to realize that there are common needs that are satisfied in a variety of ways, with no two needs being alike. Because of this, one is unable to fully interpret or supply all the requirements for the individual's well-being. Therefore, at best, a nurse can assist the individual in meeting human needs. According to Henderson, only in a dependent stage, such as in a coma or in an extreme helplessness state, is there justification in making a decision *for* the individual rather than *with* the individual.[29]

With respect to the biological concept emphasis, Henderson identifies Claude Bernard, a physiologist, and Jean Broadhurst, a microbiologist, as having an influence on her thinking.[30] Bernard's dictum of cellular physiology, the constancy of lymph system around the cell, and the emphasis on the unit structure in relationship to the laws of health provided the knowledge base of the importance of physiology.[31] From Broadhurst, Henderson was able to acquire an analytical approach to all aspects of treatment and care through participation with experiments in physiology.[32] She reports understanding that the principles of the cellular activities provided a sound basis for analyzing physiological problems. Further, Henderson states, "I believe the definition of nursing should imply an appreciation of the principle of physiological balance."[33] She also emphasizes that emotional imbalance cannot be separated from the physiological balance as these components are interrelated and each affects the other. She views mind and body as being inseparable, and thus changes in physiological function affect the emotional aspects of the individual.

The influences of two colleagues, Ida Orlando and Ernestine Wiedenbach, are incorporated in Henderson's concepts of communication and interaction. The influence of Orlando's concept of nurse-patient relationship is shown in Henderson's statement that the nurse must be sensitive to nonverbal communications and must encourage the expression of feelings.[34] The natural development of a constructive nurse-patient relationship is encouraged. Validation of need by sharing interpretation of the patient's behavior is encouraged by the use of reflective techniques. Nursing care should be provided on the basis of validated information and involves continuous observation and interpretation of patient behavior.

Wiedenbach's goal-directed and deliberative nursing approach to the individual's expressed needs for help is accepted by Henderson.[35] Henderson believes that all people have common needs; but no two patients are exactly alike, so each nurse must interpret human needs as these have meaning to the individual patient. The nurse must identify the need and supply measures that are applicable to that individual.

The concept of independent function as stated in the definition (see p. 53), indicating those activities a person could perform unaided if given the necessary strength, will, or knowledge, resulted from Henderson's experience with Dr. George C. Deaver at the Institute for the Crippled and Disabled.[36] She noted that much of the energies of the hospital personnel and of the experts in rehabilitation included the performance of activities of daily living. This experience no doubt had much influence in her viewing nursing as helping the individual to perform the activities of daily living.

HENDERSON AND THE NURSING PROCESS

Even though Henderson's definition of nursing and her explanation of it do not directly fit with the steps of the nursing process, one can see how the two concepts are related. In using Henderson's fourteen components of basic nursing care, the nurse would assess the needs of the patient based on all fourteen components. For example, in assessing the first component, "helping the patient with respiration," the nurse would gather data about the respiratory status of the patient.[37] The nurse needs to accurately observe the character of the patient's respirations. When the first component is assessed, the nurse moves to the next component and assesses the patient in relation to that component. The nurse continues gathering data about the client in relation to all the components until all fourteen are assessed. These components fit with Maslow's hierarchy of needs as explained earlier in the chapter. To gather data, the nurse uses observation, hearing, feeling, and smelling.[38] Even though Henderson does not refer directly to assessment, she implies it in her description of the fourteen components of basic nursing care.

To complete the assessment step of the nursing process, the nurse needs to analyze the data. According to Henderson, the nurse needs to have knowledge about what is normal in health and disease. Using this knowledge base, then, the nurse would compare the assessment data with what was known about that area of assessment. For example, if respirations were observed to be 40/minute in an adult aged forty, the nurse would know that this patient's respirations were elevated. Or if a patient's laboratory report showed the urine was highly concentrated, the nurse would know, "This means that the patient's fluid intake is inadequate, unless he is losing body fluids by other routes."[39] With a knowledge base, the nurse can make some sense from the assessment data. Henderson states,

> The nursing needed by the individual is affected by age, cultural background, emotional balance and his physical and intellectual capacities. All of these should be considered in the nurse's evaluation of the patient's needs for her help.[40]

By analyzing the data according to these factors, the nurse can then move into nursing diagnosis.

Henderson does not specifically discuss nursing diagnoses. She believes the physician makes the diagnosis and the nurse acts upon that diagnosis. But if one looks at Henderson's definition, it can be seen that the nursing diagnosis would deal with identifying the patient's ability to meet human needs with or without assistance, taking into consideration that person's strength, will, or knowledge. The nurse can identify actual problems such as abnormal respirations based on the assessment data and the analysis of the data, or the nurse can identify a potential problem. For example, in looking at component 11, which deals with the patient's religious practice (see p. 55), a potential problem could develop because of hospitalization and a change in the patient's normal activities of daily living.

When discussing the planning phase of nursing care, Henderson states,

> All effective nursing care is planned to some extent. A written plan forces those who make it to give some thought to the

individual's needs—unless the person's regimen is made to fit into
the routines of the institution in which he may be.[41]

She also states that the making of a plan for a patient going home,
known as *discharge planning*, is influenced by the other members of
the family.[42] Furthermore, she says that plans need to have continuing
modification, based on the patient's need. Henderson believes the
nursing care plan should be written so others giving nursing care can
follow the sequence.[43] She also emphasizes that "nursing care is
always arranged around, or fitted into, the physician's therapeutic
plan."[44] According to Henderson, the planning phase involves making
the plan fit the patient's needs, up-dating the plan as necessary based
on the patient's needs, making the plan specific so others can implement it, and making sure it fits with the physician's prescribed plan.
When writing the plan so others can implement it, the nurse is, in
effect, identifying the nursing care needs of the patient. Thus, even
though Henderson does not apply the terminology used today regarding nursing plans, she uses the concepts.

Henderson directly refers to the concept of nursing implementation. She states,

> The modification of care is the creative element which makes
> nursing an art. The basic technique, or elements of an art, can be
> described but an artistic achievement demands that the artist
> manipulate these elements in a unique arrangement. Just so each
> patient's plan of care should be different from any other.[45]

In giving this creative care, the nurse is assisting the client to perform
activities of daily living as independently as possible. The nursing care
is based on physiological principles, age, cultural background, emotional balance, and physical and intellectual capacities. Henderson
also states, "This primary function of the practicing nurse, of course,
must be performed in such a way that it promotes the physician's
therapeutic plan."[46] In other words, the nurse needs to carry out the
physician's orders of treatment.

Another important aspect of implementation that Henderson discusses is the relationship between nurse and patient. The nurse "gets
inside his skin" to better understand the patient's needs and carry out
measures to meet those needs.[47] Henderson also speaks about the
quality of care.

The quality of care is drastically affected by the preparation and native ability of the nursing personnel whether they are giving one, two, three, four, or five hours of care. Standards for "basic nursing" must therefore attempt to include at least some guiding statements on the conditions that demand more and those that demand less attention from highly qualified nurses, also to identify the aspects of care that require more or less nursing competence. The danger of turning over the physical care of the patient to relatively unqualified nurses is two-fold. They may fail to assess the patient's needs adequately but, perhaps more important, the qualified nurse, being deprived the opportunity while giving physical care to assess needs, may not find any other chance to do so. In this connection it should also be pointed out that it is easier for any person to develop an emotional supportive role with another if he can perform a tangible service.[48]

Henderson's statement supports nursing as being an interpersonal process.

This statement also shows how assessment can be used while giving care. The nursing implementation is based on helping the patient meet the fourteen components. For example, in helping the patient with the sleep and rest component, the nurse tries the known methods of inducing rest and sleep based on knowledge before giving the patient sleeping medication. In *The Nature of Nursing*, Henderson summarizes, "I see nursing as primarily complementing the patient by supplying what he needs in knowledge, will or strength to perform his daily activities and to carry out the treatment prescribed for him by the physician."[49]

Henderson bases the evaluation of each patient "according to the speed with which, or the degree to which, he performs independently the activities that make, for him, a normal day."[50] This goes back to the definition that outlines the unique function of the nurse as assisting the patient in doing those activities that person would normally perform if the necessary strength, will, and knowledge were present. To observe and measure a change, the nurse would determine how independently a patient was able to meet the fourteen components of basic nursing care. The nurse would know how independently the patient was functioning during the initial interaction. Then the nurse would compare that data to how independently the patient was functioning after the nursing plan was implemented.

To summarize the stages of the nursing process as applied to Henderson's definition of nursing and to the fourteen components of basic nursing care, refer to Table 5-1.

Table 5-1

A Summary of the Nursing Process—
Based On Henderson's Definition of Nursing

Nursing Process	
Nursing assessment	Assess needs of human being based upon the fourteen components of basic nursing care:

1. Breathing normally	8. Keep body clean and well-groomed
2. Eat and drink adequately	9. Avoid dangers in environment
3. Elimination of body wastes	10. Communication
4. Move and maintain posture	11. Worship according to one's faith
5. Sleep and rest	12. Work accomplishment
6. Suitable clothing dress/undress	13. Recreation
7. Maintain body temperature	14. Learn, discover, or satisfy curiosity

	Analysis: Compare data to knowledge base of health and disease.
Nursing diagnosis	Identify individual's ability to meet own needs with or without assistance, taking into consideration strength, will, or knowledge.
Nursing plan	Describe how the nurse can assist the individual, sick or well.
Nursing implementation	Assist the sick or well individual in the performance of activities in meeting human needs to maintain health, recover from illness, or to aid in peaceful death. Intervention based on physiological principles, age, cultural background, emotional balance, and physical and intellectual capacities. Carry out treatment prescribed by the physician.
Nursing evaluation	Based on the acceptable definition of nursing and consistent with laws related to the practice of nursing. The quality of care is drastically affected by the preparation and native ability of the nursing personnel rather than the amount of hours of care. Success of the nurse based on speed with which or degree to which patient performs independently the activities that make for a normal day.

To further illustrate the use of Henderson's fourteen components, a case study (Mr. L.) is presented in Table 5-2. Using the components as a guide, a sample nursing process is displayed. The nursing process presented demonstrates a limited example and is not intended to be an ultimate or finished process.

Table 5-2

The Nursing Process for Mr. L.
Using Henderson's Fourteen Components

Case study: Mr. L. is 25 years old, married, and the father of two preschool-age children. His wife is 6 months pregnant. Mr. L. quit school in the 10th grade. He works 16 hours a day as a skilled laborer in a factory and holds a second job washing dishes at a restaurant to meet the family expenses.

Nursing Process	*Data and Relevant Information*
Assessment	Assessment
(Assess needs of Mr. L. based on the 14 components of basic nursing care)	
1. Breathing normally.	1. Respiration rate—18, regular; smokes 2 packs of cigarettes/day; dry cough in A.M.; no shortness of breath. (Data about work environment needed.)
2. Eat and drink adequately.	2. Takes sandwich, fruit, potato chips for lunch; skips breakfast; buys soft drink; eats evening meals at the restaurant. (Results of 72-hour diet recall needed.)
3. Elimination of body wastes.	3. Reports no problems related to elimination.
4. Move and maintain posture.	4. Reports pain in both legs after 8 hours of washing dishes. No problems with mobility.
5. Sleep and rest.	5. Reports 5–6 hours sleep/night. "Feels tired most of the time."
6. Suitable clothing dress/undress.	6. Wears jeans and shirt to work—both jobs. Owns ski jacket and boots for cold weather wear. (Work environment data needed.)
7. Maintain body temperature.	7. Temperature 98.6 F. Reports no problem with being hot or cold.
8. Keep body clean and well-groomed.	8. Showers and shampoos hair daily.
9. Avoid environment hazards.	9. Wears clothes to match weather conditions. (Home environment safety—need more data.)
10. Communication.	10. Able to speak and be understood. (Communication with family—need further data.)
11. Worship according to faith.	11. Attends church (Baptist) with family every other Sunday.
12. Work accomplishment.	12. Reports happy with jobs.
13. Recreation.	13. "Need more time to spend with family."
14. Learn, discover, or satisfy curiosity.	14. Reports interested in finishing high school. Plans to pursue college education.

64

Table 5-2 *(continued)*

Nursing Process	*Data and Relevant Information*
Analysis	According to Erikson's developmental stage theory,* Mr. L. is in the intimacy stage. He is able to support his family and take care of most of their needs, except for recreational needs. Physiologically, Mr. L. is functioning within the normal range. Three concerns are: the amount of cigarettes he smokes, pains in his legs, and the inadequate sleep and rest pattern. Mr. L. plans for the future to upgrade his education and to seek better employment.
Nursing diagnosis	1. Inadequate sleep and rest pattern resulting in feeling tired and no time to spend with family. 2. Lack of knowledge regarding cigarette smoking resulting in potential health hazard. 3. Discomfort in legs resulting from standing 8 hours on the job.
Nursing plan	1. Explore with Mr. L. and wife: 　a. alternatives to working two jobs. 　b. adjust schedule to include recreation with family. 2. Determine information Mr. L. has re smoking and its hazards. 3. Formulate isometric exercises for leg pains.
Nursing implementation	Assist Mr. L. in the performance of activities in meeting his human needs to maintain health. Intervention based on physiological principles, age, cultural background, emotional balance, and physical and intellectual capacities.
Nursing evaluation	Success of the nurse based on speed with which or degree to which Mr. L. is able to carry out the activities selected.

*Erik H. Erikson, *Childhood and Society*, 2nd ed. (New York: W. W. Norton & Company, Inc., 1963), pp. 247–274.

HENDERSON AND MAN, HEALTH, SOCIETY, LEARNING, AND NURSING

In viewing the concept of man, Henderson considers the biological, psychological, sociological, and spiritual components. Her first nine components of basic nursing care reflect the physiological component, the tenth and fourteenth components speak to the psychological aspect of communicating and learning, the eleventh component reflects the spiritual aspect of religion and morals, and the twelfth and thirteenth components relate to the sociological concepts of occupation and recreation. She refers to man as having basic needs that are reflected in the fourteen components. However, she goes on to state, "It is equally important to realize that these needs are satisfied by infinitely varied patterns of living, no two of which are alike."[51] Henderson also believes that mind and body are inseparable.[52] The mind and body are interrelated, and the effects of one part are reflected in the other part.

Henderson does not emphasize the concept of society. In her writing she discusses primarily individuals. She looks at them in relation to their families but does not discuss much about the community or the impact the community has on the individual and the family. As a student her pediatric affiliation and her experience with the Visiting Nurses agency increased her concern for people. In the textbook she wrote with Harmer, she discusses the tasks of private and public agencies in keeping people healthy.[53] She believes that society wants and expects the nurse's service of acting for the patient when he is unable to function independently.[54] She also believes that

> the nurse needs the kind of education that, in our society, is only available in colleges and universities. Training programs operated on funds pinched from the budgets of service agencies cannot provide the preparation the nurse needs.[55]

This generalized education gives the nurse a better understanding of the people receiving nursing care and the various factors that influence people.

Henderson's beliefs about health are related to human functioning. She bases health on the individual's ability to function independently in relation to the fourteen components. Because good health is a challenging goal for individuals, she believes it is more difficult for the nurse to help the individual reach it.[56] She also refers to the fact the nurses tend to stress promotion of health and prevention and cure of disease.[57] Henderson explains how the factors of "age, cultural background, physical and intellectual capacities, and emotional balance affect one's health."[58]

Henderson's fourteenth component deals with the concept of learning. She believes the nurse needs to assist the individual to "learn, discover, or satisfy the curiosity that leads to 'normal' development and health."[59] She believes patients learn by the examples the nurse gives to them and by the answers the nurse offers to their questions. Henderson subscribes to the concept of sequential learning, as follows. First, beginning nursing students learn the classroom material. Then they observe care given by expert practitioners during practice in the laboratory. Next the students work with experienced nurses by being assigned to the patients under these nurses' care. Finally, the students function independently in giving basic aspects of nursing care. Based on her experience as a student, Henderson believes it is important for students to see their teachers practicing nursing. She feels this experience would have greatly enhanced her own learning. Henderson discusses the development of inquiring minds and problem-solving techniques. She relates these ideas to how students should be taught in order to develop in this manner.

Henderson supports life-long learning and states, "If the student is to acquire the ability as a graduate to continually increase her clinical competence, she should begin to practice independent study as an undergraduate."[60] She also believes that teachers "can create an atmosphere conducive to learning and can help the student develop the habit of study which, if continued as a graduate, will lead to ever-increasing nursing competence."[61] The teacher has the responsibility for an environment conducive to learning, and the learner has the responsibility to read, to study, and to learn.

Henderson's view of the concept of nursing is interesting from the time perspective of her writings. She believes nurses need a liberalized education to gain knowledge about the sciences, social sciences, and humanities. The nurse's practice is based on Henderson's definition of nursing and the fourteen components of basic nursing care and carrying out the physician's therapeutic plan. The creative implementation of nursing care makes the care individualized for each patient. It is the nurse's responsibility to improve patient care through nursing research.

> The nurse who operates under a definition that specifies an area
> of independent practice, or an area of expertness, must assume

responsibility for identifying problems, for continually validating her function, for improving the methods she uses, and for measuring the effect of nursing care. In this era research is the name we attach to the most reliable type of analysis.[62]

Figure 5-1 illustrates the main concepts of Henderson's definition of nursing. It demonstrates nursing as assisting the sick and well individual to perform those activities contributing to health, recovery of health, or peaceful death. Figure 5-1 also identifies nursing as assisting individuals in becoming independent as soon as possible in the performance of the activities of daily living. Furthermore, to help an individual perform activities unaided, the nurse needs to consider that person's strength, knowledge, and will.

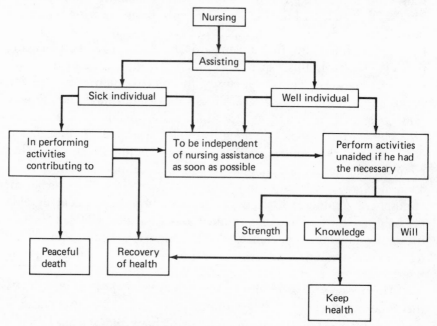

Figure 5-1. Conceptualization of Henderson's definition of nursing. [*Modified from* Nursing Development Conference Group, *Concept Formalization in Nursing Process and Product* (Boston: Little, Brown & Company, 1973), p. 56. Used with permission.]

LIMITATIONS

Although Henderson based her ideas about nursing care on the fundamental human needs and the physical and emotional aspects of the individual, the concept of the holistic nature of human beings does not emerge. For example, the fact that a person's oxygenation needs will have an effect on the other remaining components of basic nursing care is unclear. Also, if an assumption can be made that the fourteen components are prioritized, it is of significance to note there is an interrelationship among the components since each component does affect the next one on the list. If priority according to individual needs is implied in the listing of the components, does the presenting emotional problem take a back seat to physical care, and is this area of care deferred until such time the physiological need areas are given proper attention? Henderson specifies that the nurse must consider such factors as age, temperament, social or cultural status, and physical and intellectual capacity in the use of the components, thus emphasizing differences in the individual but not necessarily the interrelationship of these factors. However, the reader must keep in mind Henderson wrote her ideas about nursing before the emergence of the concept of holism.

The fact that the majority of the fourteen components are focused on the physiological needs gives the impression that nursing care considerations are more on the physical than the psychosocial needs. This is not to say there must be a balance, but a misunderstanding that nursing care emphasis is more on the physical aspects than on the psychosocial aspects may be a possible conclusion.

In assisting the individual in the dying process, Henderson acknowledges that the nurse helps, but there is little explanation as to what is done in this area. In her statement of the definition of nursing, the placing of a parenthesis around the, words *peaceful death* brings questions as to why this was done.

CONCLUSIONS

The concept of nursing presented by Henderson in her definition of nursing and the fourteen components is self-explanatory. Therefore, it could be used as a guide by most without difficulty. Many of Henderson's thoughts and ideas continue to be useful today. This can be validated by the demand of her ICN publication, which in 1972 was in its seventh printing.

If a suggestion to improve Henderson's concept of nursing can be made, the incorporation of holism and system theory may provide a clearer explanation of the relationship of the components. Also confirmation of the priority listing of the components is needed to clarify what the nurse is to do if the presenting problem is other than a physical one.

When one considers the time in which Henderson wrote about her ideas and beliefs about nursing, she deserves much credit as one of the pioneers giving direction to the development of nursing theories.

SUMMARY

Henderson states,

> I believe that the function the nurse performs is primarily an independent one—that of acting for the patient when he lacks knowledge, physical strength, or the will to act for himself as he would ordinarily act in health, or in carrying out prescribed therapy. The function is seen as complex and creative, as offering unlimited opportunity for the application of the physical, biological, and social sciences, and the development of skills based on them.[63]

The fourteen components of basic nursing care are viewed by Henderson as the unique function of the nurse. This together with her definition of nursing provides the basis for nursing practice.

NOTES

1. Virginia Henderson, *The Nature of Nursing* (New York: The Macmillan Company, 1966); idem, *Basic Principles of Nursing Care* (Geneva: International Council of Nurses, 1972).
2. Henderson, *The Nature of Nursing*, p. 1.
3. Ibid., p. 6.
4. Ibid.
5. Ibid., p. 7.
6. Ibid., p. 9.
7. Ibid., p. 10.
8. Ibid.
9. Bertha Harmer and Virginia Henderson, *Textbook of the Principles and Practice of Nursing*, 4th ed. (New York: The Macmillan Company, 1939); Gwendolyn Safier, *Contemporary American Leaders in Nursing* (New York: McGraw-Hill Book Company, 1977), p. 119.
10. Henderson, *The Nature of Nursing*, p. 3.

11. Ibid.
12. "ANA Statement on Auxiliary Personnel in Nursing Service," *The American Journal of Nursing*, 62, no. 7 (1962).
13. Bertha Harmer, *Textbook of the Principles and Practice of Nursing* (New York: The Macmillan Company, 1922), p. 3; Nursing Development Conference Group, *Concept Formalization in Nursing: Process and Product* (Boston: Little, Brown & Company, 1973), p. 40.
14. Bertha Harmer and Virginia Henderson, *Textbook of Principles and Practice of Nursing*, 5th ed. (New York: The Macmillan Company, 1955), p. 4; Nursing Development Conference Group, *Concept Formalization*, pp. 41-42.
15. Harmer, *Textbook*, p. 4; Nursing Development Conference Group, *Concept Formalization*, p. 41.
16. Henderson, *The Nature of Nursing*, pp. 16-17.
17. Ibid., p. 15.
18. Ibid.
19. Ibid.
20. Ibid., p. 16.
21. Henderson, *Basic Principles*, p. 3.
22. Henderson, *The Nature of Nursing*, p. 16.
23. Ibid., p. 11.
24. Ibid.
25. Henderson, *Basic Principles*, p. 7.
26. Abraham Maslow, *Motivation and Personality* (New York: Harper & Row Publishers, Inc., 1954); and Marjorie Byrne and Lida Thompson, *Key Concepts for the Study and Practice of Nursing* (St. Louis, Mo.: The C. V. Mosby Co., 1972), p. 10.
27. Ibid.
28. Henderson, *Basic Principles*, p. 7.
29. Ibid.
30. Henderson, *The Nature of Nursing*, p. 10.
31. Ibid.
32. Ibid.
33. Ibid., p. 11.
34. Ida Jean Orlando, *The Dynamic Nurse-Patient Relationship, Function, Process and Principles* (New York: G. P. Putnam's Sons, 1961), p. 91; and Henderson, *The Nature of Nursing*, p. 14.
35. Ernestine Wiedenbach, *Clinical Nursing: A Helping Art* (New York: Springer Publishing Co., Inc., 1964), p. 118; and Henderson, *The Nature of Nursing*, p. 15.
36. Henderson, *The Nature of Nursing*, p. 12.
37. Henderson, *Basic Principles*, p. 19.
38. Ibid., p. 41.
39. Ibid., p. 25.

40. Ibid., p. 10.
41. Ibid., p. 14.
42. Ibid.
43. Ibid.
44. Ibid., p. 15.
45. Ibid., p. 14.
46. Henderson, *The Nature of Nursing*, p. 27.
47. Ibid., p. 24.
48. Henderson, *Basic Principles*, p. 13.
49. Henderson, *The Nature of Nursing*, p. 21.
50. Ibid., p. 30.
51. Henderson, *Basic Principles*, p. 7.
52. Henderson, *The Nature of Nursing*, p. 11.
53. Harmer and Henderson, *Textbook of the Principles*, p. 33.
54. Henderson, *The Nature of Nursing*, p. 68.
55. Ibid., p. 69.
56. Henderson, *Basic Principles*, p. 5.
57. Henderson, *The Nature of Nursing*, pp. 21-22.
58. Henderson, *Basic Principles*, p. 10.
59. Ibid., p. 13.
60. Henderson, *The Nature of Nursing*, p. 46.
61. Ibid., p. 48.
62. Henderson, *Basic Principles*, p. 38.
63. Henderson, *The Nature of Nursing*, p. 68.

6

HILDEGARD E. PEPLAU

Janice Ryan Belcher and Lois J. Brittain Fish

Hildegard Peplau was born in Reading, Pennsylvania, on September 1, 1909. Dr. Peplau graduated from a diploma program in nursing in Pottstown, Pennsylvania, in 1931. She graduated from Bennington College in 1943 with a B.A. in Interpersonal Psychology and from Columbia University in New York in 1947 with a M.A. in Psychiatric Nursing and in 1953 with an Ed.D. in Curriculum Development. Dr. Peplau's nursing experience includes private and general duty hospital experience, two years in the U.S. Army, nursing research, and part-time private practice in psychiatric nursing. She has taught graduate psychiatric nursing for many years and is a retired professor emeritus from Rutgers University. Dr. Peplau spent two years in Belgium facilitating the first postbaccalaureate nursing program in central Europe.

Hildegard Peplau published the book Interpersonal Relations in Nursing *in 1952.[1] She has also published numerous articles in professional magazines on topics ranging from interpersonal concepts to current issues in nursing. Her pamphlet "Basic Principles of Patient Counseling" was derived from her research and workshops.[2]*

Dr. Peplau has served with many organizations including the World Health Organization, National Institute of Mental Health, and the Nurse Corps. She is past Executive Director and President of the American Nurses' Association. She has served as a nursing consultant to various foreign countries and to the Surgeon General of the Air Force. Her many contributions to nursing are the result of her pioneer qualities in communicating her perceptions concerning nursing.

Hildegard Peplau's book *Interpersonal Relations in Nursing* will be considered as the reference source for her nursing theory. In 1952 Peplau published this book, referring to it as a "partial theory for the practice of nursing."[3] In the book, Peplau discusses the phases of the interpersonal process, roles in nursing situations, and methods for studying nursing as an interpersonal process. This chapter defines the crux of her nursing theory to be the phases of the interpersonal process and relates the other ideas to this central core.

Theories of nursing usually evolve around the four concepts of humanity, health, society, and nursing. Peplau defines man* as an organism who "strives in its own way to reduce tension generated by needs."[4] Health is defined as "a word symbol that implies forward movement of personality and other ongoing human processes in the direction of creative, constructive, productive, personal, and community living."[5] Society is not mentioned as such, but Peplau does encourage nursing to consider culture and mores when the patient changes environments, for example, when the patient adjusts to the hospital routine.[6] Peplau's lack of a clear definition of society comes from her focus on the specific nurse/patient relationship. Because of this focus, the fourth concept, nursing, is expanded, and the underlying principles of the interpersonal process are explored more fully.

Hildegard Peplau considers nursing a "significant therapeutic, interpersonal process."[7] She defines it as a "human relationship between an individual who is sick, or in need of health services, and a nurse especially educated to recognize and to respond to the need for help."[8]

Nursing is therapeutic in that it is a healing art, assisting an individual who is sick or in need of health care. It can be viewed as an interpersonal process because it involves interaction between two or more individuals with a common goal. In nursing, this common goal provides the incentive for the therapeutic process in which the nurse and patient respect each other as individuals, both of them learning and growing as a result of the interaction. Learning takes place when

---

*Peplau uses *man* and *he* in the generic sense.

an individual selects stimuli in an environment and develops more fully as a result of reactions to these stimuli.[9]

The attainment of this goal, or any goal, is achieved through the use of a series of steps following a certain pattern. As the relationship of the nurse to patient develops in this therapeutic pattern, there is flexibility in the way in which the nurse functions in practice—by making judgments, by utilizing skills founded in scientific knowledge, by utilizing technical abilities, and by assuming roles.

When the nurse and patient first identify a problem and begin to focus on a course of action, they approach this path from diverse backgrounds and individual uniqueness. One might view each individual as being composed of a biological-psychological-spiritual-sociological structure, one that will not react the same as any other. Each individual has learned differently from the distinct environment, mores, customs, and beliefs of that individual's given culture. Each individual comes with preconceived ideas that influence perceptions, and it is these differences in perception that are so important in the interpersonal process. In addition, the nurse, from an educational background, contributes an understanding of developmental theories, of concepts of life's adaptations, and of conflict responses, as well as a greater insight of nursing's professional role in the interpersonal process. As nurse and patient continue the relationship, an understanding of one another's roles and the factors surrounding the problem increases until both nurse and patient are mutually sharing in a collaborative manner toward resolution of the problem.

The nurse and the patient work together in seeking the solution to the patient's problem, and as a result both become more knowledgeable and mature in the process. Peplau also views nursing as a "maturing force" and an "educative instrument."[10] She feels nursing is a learning experience of oneself as well as of the other individual involved in the interpersonal action. This concept is supported by Genevieve Burton, another nursing author from the 1950s, who states, "Behavior of others must be understood in light of self understanding."[11] Thus, one who is more in touch with oneself would be more aware of the various types of reactions induced in another individual.

As the nurse guides the patient toward the solutions of the everyday encounters, the methods and principles utilized in the professional practice become increasingly more effective. Each encounter influences the nurse's personal and professional development. Thus, the kind of person the nurse becomes has a direct influence on the therapeutic, interpersonal relationship.

Peplau identifies four sequential phases in interpersonal relation-ships: (1) *orientation,* (2) *identification,* (3) *exploitation,* and (4) *resolu-tion.* Each phase will be discussed and related to the nursing process. These phases are very important as viewed in the nursing process used in nursing today. Each of these phases overlaps and interrelates as the process evolves toward a solution. Different nursing roles are assumed during the various phases.

These roles can be broadly described in the following manner:

Teacher: One who imparts knowledge in reference to a need or interest.

Resource: One who provides specific, needed information that aids in the understanding of a problem or new situation.

Counselor: One who, through the use of certain skills and attitudes, aids another in recognizing, facing, ac-cepting, and resolving problems that are interfering with the other person's ability to live happily and effectively.

Leader: One who carries out the process of initiation and maintenance of group goals through interaction.

Technical expert: One who provides physical care by displaying clin-ical skills and has the ability to operate equipment in this care.

Surrogate: One who takes the place of another.

PEPLAU'S PHASES IN NURSING

Orientation

In the initial phase of *orientation* the nurse and patient meet as two strangers. The patient and/or the family has a "felt need";[12] therefore professional assistance is sought. This need may not be readily identified or understood by those individuals who are involved. For example, a sixteen-year-old girl may call the community mental health center just because she feels "very down." It is in this phase that the nurse needs to assist the patient and family in realizing what is happening to the patient.

It is of the utmost importance that the nurse work collaboratively with the patient and family in analyzing the situation, so that they (together) recognize, can clarify and define the existing problem. Take the previous example: The nurse, in the counselor role, may help the teen-age girl who feels "very down" to realize that these feelings may be the result of an argument with her mother this morning over last evening's date. As the nurse continues to listen to the girl, there may be a pattern established between arguing with her mother and feeling depressed. As these feelings are discussed, the girl may recognize the arguing as the precipitating factor that causes the depression. Thus the nurse and the patient have defined the problem. Then, the daughter and the parents agree to discuss the concern with the nurse. By mutually clarifying and defining the problem in the orientation phase, the patient directs the accumulated energy from the anxiety of unmet needs to more constructively dealing with the presenting problem. Rapport is continually being established while concerns are being identified.

While the patient and family are talking to the nurse, a mutual decision needs to be made regarding what type of professional assistance should be pursued. The nurse, as a resource person, may work with the patient and family. As an alternative the nurse might, upon mutual agreement of all parties involved, refer the family to another source such as a psychologist or social worker. In the orientation phase, the nurse, patient, and family plan what type of services are needed.

The orientation phase is directly affected by the patient's and nurse's attitudes about giving or receiving aid from a reciprocal person. Therefore, in this beginning phase, the nurse needs to be aware of personal reactions to the patient. For example, the nurse may react differently to the forty-year-old man with abdominal pain who enters the emergency room quietly than to the forty-year-old man with a history of regular alcohol abuse who enters the emergency room boisterously after a few drinks. The nurse's, as well as the patient's, culture, religion, race, educational background, past experiences, and preconceived ideas play a part in the nurse's reaction to the patient. The same influencing factors play a part in the patient's reaction to the nurse. For example, the patient may have stereotyped the nurse into performing only technical skills such as giving medications or taking blood pressures and therefore may not have perceived the nurse as the resource person who can help define the problem. Nursing is an interpersonal process, and both the patient and nurse have an equally important part in the therapeutic interaction.

The nurse, the patient, and the family work together to recognize, clarify, and define the existing problem. This in turn decreases the tension and anxiety associated with the "felt need"[13] and the fear of the unknown. Decreasing tension and anxiety prevents future problems that might arise as a result of repressing an event. Stressful situations are identified through therapeutic conversation. It is imperative that the patient work through personal feelings connected with the events leading up to an illness.

Thus, in the beginning of the orientation phase, the nurse and the patient meet as strangers. At the end of the orientation phase they are concurrently striving to identify the problem and are becoming more comfortable with one another. The patient is settling into the helping environment. The nurse and the patient are now ready to logically progress to the next phase.

Identification

The next phase, referred to as *identification*, is one in which the patient responds selectively to people who can meet his needs. Each patient responds differently in this phase. The patient might actively seek the nurse out or stoically wait until the nurse seeks him out. The response to the nurse is threefold: (1) participate with and be interdependent with the nurse, (2) be autonomous and independent from the nurse; or (3) be passive and dependent on the nurse.[14] An example would be that of a seventy-year-old man who wants to plan his new 1600 calorie diabetic diet. If the relationship is interdependent, the nurse and patient collaborate on the meal planning. Should the relationship be independent, the patient would plan the diet himself with minimal input from the nurse. In a dependent relationship, the nurse does the meal planning for the patient.

Throughout the identification phase, both the patient and nurse must clarify each other's perceptions and expectations.[15] Past experiences of both the patient and the nurse will have a bearing on what their expectations will be during this interpersonal process. As mentioned in the orientation phase, the initial attitudes of the patient and the nurse are important in building a working relationship for identifying the problem and deciding on appropriate assistance.

The perception and expectations of the patient and nurse in the identification phase are even more complex than in the preceding phase. The patient is now responding to the helper selectively. This requires a more intense relationship. To illustrate, a patient may mention to the nurse her inability to understand the arm exercises that have been previously explained to her as an important regimen following her mastectomy (breast removal). The nurse observes the affected arm to be edematous (swollen). The patient admits not doing her arm exercises while the nurse explores possible reasons for the edema. In order to facilitate the patient's understanding and subsequent resumption of the exercises, the nurse identifies professional people, such as the physical therapist, the nurse, and the physician, who can clarify the patient's misconceptions. At this time, the patient states that she does not care to discuss the exercises with the nurse or physical therapist because she perceives only the physician as having the necessary information. Thus, previous perceptions of nursing and physical therapy influence the patient's current decision on the selection of a professional person.

While working through this identification phase, the patient begins to have a feeling of belonging and a capability of dealing with the problem, which decreases her feelings of helplessness and hopelessness. This in turn creates an optimistic attitude from which inner strength ensues.

Exploitation

Following identification, the patient moves into the *exploitation* phase in which advantage of all available services is taken. The degree to which these services are utilized is based on the interests and needs of the patient. The individual begins to feel an integral part of the helping environment. She/he feels as though some control over the situation is gained by extracting help from the services offered. Take the example of the woman with the edematous arm. During this phase the patient begins to absorb the information given to her for the arm exercises. She reads pamphlets and watches a film describing the exercises; she discusses questions with the nurse; and she may inquire about starting an exercise group through the physical therapy department.

During this phase some patients may make more demands than they did when they were seriously ill. They may make many minor requests or may apply other "attention-getting" techniques depending on their individual needs. These actions may often be difficult, if not impossible, for the health care provider to completely understand. The nurse must deal with the unconscious forces causing the patient's actions. The principles of interviewing techniques must be used in order to understand and adequately deal with the underlying problems. It is important that the nurse explore the possible causes for the patient's behavior. A therapeutic relationship must be maintained by conveying an attitude of acceptance, concern, and trust. The nurse must encourage the patient to recognize and explore feelings, thoughts, emotions, and behaviors by providing a nonjudgmental atmosphere and therapeutic emotional climate.

Some patients may take an active interest in, and become involved in, self-care. Such a patient will become more self-sufficient and will demonstrate initiative by establishing appropriate behavior for goal attainment. Through self-determination, the patient progressively develops responsibility for self, belief in potentialities, and adjustment toward self-reliance and independence. These patients realistically begin to establish their own goals toward improved health status. They strive to achieve a pattern or direction to their lives and a feeling of wellness. This is accomplished by becoming productive, by trusting and depending on their own capabilities, and by becoming responsible for their own actions, thus becoming more fully themselves. As a result, as their unique personality continues to form, they develop sources of inner strength with which to face new problems or challenges.

Most patients fluctuate between dependence on others, as in the impaired health role, and the independence of functioning at an optimal health level. Using the previous example, this patient may want to actively exercise on schedule one day but will state she is too tired the next day. The nurse then needs to take the initiative to remind the patient of her scheduled exercises. This type of intermittent behavior can be compared to the adjustment reaction of the adolescent or a dependency-independency conflict. The patient may temporarily be in a dependent role while the simultaneous need for independence exists. Various causes may trigger the onset of this emotional disequilibrium. The patient will vacillate unpredictably between the two states. She/he will appear confused and anxious, protesting dependence while fearing independence. In caring for patients who fluctuate between dependence and independence, the nurse must deal with the particular behavior presented rather than attempting to handle the composite problem of inconsistency. The nurse must provide an atmosphere that carries no threat, one in which a person can face himself, recognize his weaknesses, use his strengths without imposing them on others, and accept help from others. The nurse must also be fully aware of the various facets of communication including clarifying, listening, accepting, and interpreting. Correct use of all these factors will assist the patient to meet his challenges and will pave the way toward maximum wholesome adjustment. Thus, the nurse aids the patient in exploiting all avenues of help, and progress is made toward the final step—the resolution phase.

Resolution

The last phase of Peplau's interpersonal process is *resolution*. The patient's needs have already been met by the collaborative efforts of the nurse and patient. Now, the patient and nurse must terminate their therapeutic relationship and must dissolve the links between them.

Sometimes dissolving these links is very strenuous for both the patient and the nurse. Dependency needs in a therapeutic relationship often continue on psychologically after the physiological needs are met. The patient may feel that it "is just not time yet" to end the relationship. For example, a new mother has a desire to learn to take her baby's temperature. During the first home visit the public health nurse and the new mother set their goal of having the mother take the baby's temperature correctly. After instruction and demonstration by the public health nurse on the first visit, the mother takes the temperature correctly on the second visit. Their goal is met. The relationship is ended because the mother's problem was solved. However, one week after the resolution, the mother telephones the public health nurse three times concerning minor questions on infant care. The mother at this point has not dissolved the dependency link with the public health nurse.

The final resolution may also be strenuous for the nurse. In the above example, the mother may be willing to terminate the relationship, but the public health nurse may continue to visit the home to see how the baby is doing. The nurse may be unable to become free of this bond in their relationship. In resolution, as in the other phases, anxiety and tension will increase in the patient and in the nurse if there is unsuccessful completion of the phase.

During successful resolution, the patient drifts away from identifying with the helping person, the nurse. This phase is a direct outgrowth of the successful completion of the other phases. The patient breaks the bond with the nurse. The patient's collaborative efforts are not independent efforts, and a healthier emotional balance is demonstrated. The nurse also must establish independence from the patient. When the dissolving of the therapeutic interpersonal process is sequential to the previous phases, the patient and the nurse both become stronger maturing individuals. The patient's needs are met and movement can be made toward new goals.

RELATIONSHIP BETWEEN PEPLAU'S PHASES AND THE NURSING PROCESS

Peplau's continuum of the four phases of *orientation, identification, exploitation,* and *resolution* can be compared to the nursing process as discussed in Chapter 2. The nursing process in Chapter 2 is defined as "a deliberate, intellectual activity whereby the practice of nursing is approached in an orderly, systematic manner."*

There are basic similarities between the nursing process and Peplau's interpersonal phases. Both Peplau's phases and the nursing process are sequential and focus on therapeutic interactions. Both utilize problem-solving techniques for the nurse and patient to collaborate on, with the end purpose of meeting the patient's needs. Both go from general to specific, for example, the patient's vague feelings to specific facts concerning the vague feelings. And both include observation, communication, and recording as basic tools utilized by nursing.

There are differences, too, between Peplau's phases and the nursing process. When considering differences, it must be taken into account that Peplau's book *Interpersonal Relations in Nursing* was published in 1952. Professional nursing today is functioning with more defined goals. Movement is away from the nurse as the physician's helper and more toward the nurse as a consumer advocate. For instance, today part of the nursing process is a nursing diagnosis. The American Nurses' Association, in the *Standards of Nursing Practice,* states: "Nursing diagnoses are derived from health status data."[16] Peplau, however, stated (in 1952) that the physician's primary function was "recognizing the full impact of the patient's nuclear problem and the kind of professional assistance that is needed," which results, for the physician, in "the task of evaluating and diagnosing emergent problems."[17] This is in opposition to the present recognition of the independent nursing function.

*See p. 12.

Nursing functions, according to Peplau, include clarification of the information the physician gives the patient as well as collection of data about the patient that may point out other problem areas.[18] Today, however, with nursing's expanded roles, we have independent nurse practitioners who may or may not refer the patient to the physician, depending on the patient's need. Through expanded roles such as this, nursing is becoming more accountable and responsible, giving professional nursing greater legal independence. The nursing process provides a mode for evaluating the quality of nursing care rendered, which is the core of legal accountability.

Communication techniques are more analytical as a result of increased nursing research and social science research. In the 1950s Ludwig von Bertalanffy abstracted the general system theory. This theory takes into account interrelationships between parts and the whole, and has vast implications for nursing.[19] Through the development of this theory, nursing can be seen as viewing the interactions between the patient and his environment. Substantiating this, nursing theorist Martha Rogers, using general system theory, discussed the need of nursing to recognize, "the complementary nature of the man-environment relationship."[20]

Peplau gives the variables in nursing situations as needs, frustration, conflict, and anxiety. She further relates that these variables must be dealt with for growth to occur, as the nurse facilitates healthy development of each personality. It is readily seen that Peplau was influenced by some of the theories of the time, especially Harry S. Sullivan's interpersonal theory[21] and Sigmund Freud's theory of psychodynamics.[22]

In nursing today, variables such as intrafamily dynamics, socioeconomic forces (e.g., financial resources), personal space considerations, and community social service resources should be taken into account for each patient. These variables provide a broader perspective for viewing nursing situations instead of considering only the personal factors of needs, frustration, conflict, and anxiety. Currently, even a family, a group, or a community may be collectively defined as the patient.

Nursing has also broadened its perspective in helping the patient reach a fuller health potential through a greater emphasis on health maintenance and promotion. Martha Rogers states, "Maintenance and promotion of health, prevention of disease, nursing diagnosis, intervention, and rehabilitation encompass the scope of nursing's goals."[23]

Nurses are actively seeking to identify health problems in a variety of community and institutional settings today.

The specific components of the nursing process and Peplau's phases will now be discussed. Peplau's orientation phase parallels the beginning of the *assessment phase* in that both the nurse and patient come together as strangers. This meeting is initiated by the patient who expresses a need, although the need is not always understood. Conjointly, the nurse and patient begin to work through recognizing, clarifying, and defining facts related to this need. This step is presently referred to as the data collection in the assessment phase of the nursing process.

In the nursing process the need is not necessarily a "felt need."[24] For example, the nurse may be currently functioning in the community by doing health assessments of people who perceive themselves to be healthy. The school nurse may do hearing screening for school children. If a hearing deficit is discovered, a referral is initiated by the nurse. The children do not usually seek out the nurse for this deficit. In this situation, the need must be identified for the child and for his parents in order to persuade them to seek assistance regarding the hearing deficit. Supplying the data on a note sent home to the parents might precipitate the parents' and child's perception of the need. This is congruent with the first part of Edgar H. Schein's model of change, the unfreezing of the established equilibrium so change can take place. Schein states, "If change is to occur, therefore, it must be preceded by an alteration of the present stable equilibrium which supports the present behavior and attitudes."[25] Supplying the data would be one stimulus for change. The nurse may also have to follow up the child's note with a telephone call or a home visit and additional data such as poor grades in order to facilitate the family's entry into the unfreezing stage or into Peplau's "felt need" phase of orientation.[26]

Orientation and nursing assessment are not synonymous and must not be confused. Collecting data is continuous throughout Peplau's phases. In the nursing process, the initial collection of data is the nursing assessment, and further collection of data becomes an integral part of reassessment (see Chapter 2, Figure 2-1).

The *nursing diagnosis* evolves once the health problems or deficits are identified. The nursing diagnosis is a summary statement of the data collected. It delineates the patient's problem or potential problem. Peplau states that "during the period of orientation the patient clarifies his first whole impression of his problem";[27] whereas, in the nursing process, the nurse's judgment forms the nursing diagnosis from the data collected.

Mutually set patient and nursing goals evolve from the nursing diagnosis. These goals give direction to the plan and indicate the appropriate helping resources. When helping resources are discussed, the patient then can selectively identify with the helpers. According to Peplau, the patient is viewed as being in the identification phase.

When the nurse and patient collaborate on goals, there may be a clash based on the preconceptions and expectations of each person, as described earlier in Peplau's identification phase. These discrepancies must be resolved before mutually stated goals can be agreed on. Goal setting should be an interdependent action between nurse and patient.

In the *planning* component of the nursing process, the nurse must specifically formulate how the patient is going to achieve the mutually set goals. In this step the nurse considers the patient's own skills for handling his personal problems. Peplau stresses that the nurse wants to develop a therapeutic relationship so that the patient's anxiety is channeled constructively to seeking resources, thus decreasing feelings of hopelessness. This step in planning can still be considered within Peplau's identification phase.

The patient also begins to have a feeling of belonging because of mutual respect, communication, and interest. The feeling of belonging must be analyzed and should be a thrust toward a healthier personality and not imitative behavior.[28] Peplau states, "Some patients identify too readily with nurses, expecting that all of their wants will be taken care of and that nothing will be expected of them."[29] In Peplau's identification phase, the patient selectively responds to people who can meet his personal needs. Therefore, the identification phase is patient-initiated.

The planning stage of the nursing process gives direction and meaning to the nursing action toward resolving the patient's problems. The nurse utilizes the knowledge from her/his educational background to scientifically base the plan of nursing action.

In *implementation*, as in exploitation, the patient is finally reaping benefits from the therapeutic relationship by drawing on the nurse's knowledge and expertise. In both stages (implementation and exploitation) the individualized plans have already been formed, based on the patient's interest and needs. Therefore, in both stages the plans are initiated toward completion of desired goals. There is a difference, however, between exploitation, where the patient is the one who

actively seeks varying types of services in obtaining the maximal benefits available, and implementation, where there is a prescribed plan or
procedure, holistic in nature, to achieve mutually predetermined goals
or objectives based on the nurse's intellectual knowledge and technical
skills. Exploitation is patient-oriented, whereas implementation can be
accomplished by the client or by other persons including health professionals and the client's family.

In Peplau's resolution stage the other phases have been successfully worked through, the needs have been met, and resolution
and termination are the end result. Although Peplau does not discuss
evaluation per se, evaluation is an inherent factor in determining the
status of readiness for the patient to proceed through the resolution
phase.

In the nursing process the evaluation is a separate step, and
mutually established expected end behaviors are utilized as tools for
evaluation. Time limits on attainment of these behaviors are set for
the purposes of evaluation, although these limits need not be adhered
to strictly. Circumstances may arise that require an adjustment on the
time constraints.

In evaluation, if the situation is clear-cut, the problem moves
toward termination. However, if the problem is unresolved, goals and
objectives are not met; and if care is ineffective, a reassessment must
be done. New goals, planning, and implementation are then established.

PEPLAU'S PHASES RELATED
AS A THEORY

Peplau's interpersonal approach to nursing has the characteristics of a
theory. As discussed in Chapter 1, theories logically interrelate concepts and are consistent with other theories, laws, and principles. Also,
theories must add to the general body of knowledge of a discipline,
thus improving practice. In addition, theories must be able to be
tested.

The phases of orientation, identification, exploitation, and resolution progress logically in nature, interrelating the different components of each phase. It can be seen that Peplau broadly relates these
four phases to the interpersonal concepts of humanity, health, society,
and nursing. For example, in the phase of orientation there are the
components of nurse, patient, strangers, problems, and anxiety.

Peplau's phases are consistent with other theories such as Maslow's need theory[30] and Selye's stress theory.[31] General system theory could be broadly related to the four phases. For instance, the nurse and patient could each be defined as a system with the interaction of the four phases being energy exchanges of input, throughput, and output of each nurse and patient system.

Peplau's work has contributed greatly to the body of knowledge not only in psychiatric-mental health nursing but in nursing in general. Today, nursing is still defined as an interpersonal process. Also, communication and interviewing skills are basic tools of nursing.

With regard to Peplau's contribution to research in psychiatric-mental health nursing, Professor Grayce Sills states that in the 1950s two-thirds of research was concentrated on relationships.[32] Dr. Sills says, "At Teachers College, Columbia University, Peplau's (1952) work influenced the interpersonal nature and direction of clinical work and studies."[33] Presently, as in the past, researchers are attempting to test Peplau's theory. However, there are drawbacks in testing hypotheses based on interpersonal processes as in any of the social science fields dealing with human behaviors.

SUMMARY

The text *Interpersonal Relations in Nursing*, published in 1952, is still applicable in theory and practice. The interpersonal process is indeed an integral part of present-day nursing. The core of Peplau's theory of nursing is the interpersonal process. This process consists of the sequential phases of orientation, identification, exploitation, and resolution. These phases overlap, interrelate, and vary in time duration. The nurse and patient first clarify the patient's problem, and mutual expectations and goals are explored while deciding on appropriate plans for improved health status. This process is influenced by both the nurse's and patient's perceptions and preconceived ideas emerging from their individual uniqueness.

Both Peplau's phases and the nursing process are sequential and focus on therapeutic interactions. Through mutual exploration of the patient's difficulty and the nurse-patient relationship, a broader understanding of the patient's problem and new alternative approaches toward reaching the solution are uncovered.

When two persons meet in a creative relationship, there is a continuing sense of mutuality and togetherness throughout the experience. Both individuals are involved in a process of self-fulfillment. This process becomes a growth experience.

Peplau focuses on a specific nurse and patient relationship. Today's nursing process, however, may view the patient collectively as a group, family, or community. Thus, today's nursing process takes the total environment more into account.

Peplau's nursing theory, the interpersonal process, has as its foundation, theories of interaction. It has contributed to nursing in the areas of clinical practice, theory, and research, adding to today's nursing knowledge base. Thus, Peplau's theory has facilitated increased understanding of the patterns of interactions and the nurse/patient value systems, giving fuller resources from which nurses can draw for future encounters with patients who have similar needs.

NOTES

1. Hildegard E. Peplau, *Interpersonal Relations in Nursing* (New York: G. P. Putnam's Sons, 1952).
2. Hildegard E. Peplau, "Basic Principles of Patient Counseling," n.d.; and "Profile: Hildegard E. Peplau, R.N., Ed.D.," *Nursing '74*, 4, no. 2 (February 1974), 13.
3. Peplau, *Interpersonal Relations*, p. 261.
4. Ibid., p. 82.
5. Ibid., p. 12.
6. Ibid., p. 28.
7. Ibid., p. 16.
8. Ibid., pp. 5-6.
9. Ibid., p. 35.
10. Ibid., p. 8.
11. Genevieve Burton, *Personal, Impersonal, and Interpersonal: A Guide for Nurses* (New York: Springer New York, Inc., 1958), p. 7.
12. Peplau, *Interpersonal Relations*, p. 18.
13. Ibid.
14. Ibid., p. 33.
15. Ibid., p. 36.
16. Congress for Nursing Practice, *Standards of Nursing Practice* (Kansas City, Mo.: American Nurses' Association, 1973), p. 2.
17. Peplau, *Interpersonal Relations*, p. 23.
18. Ibid.
19. Ludwig von Bertalanffy, *Main Currents in Modern Thought*, cited by Mary Elizabeth Hazzard, in "An Overview of Systems Theory," *Nursing Clinics of North America*, 6 no. 3 (September 1971), 385.

20. Martha E. Rogers, An Introduction to the Theoretical Basis of Nursing (Philadelphia: F. A. Davis Company, 1970), p. 85.
21. Harry S. Sullivan, Conceptions of Modern Psychiatry (Washington, D.C: William Alanson White Psychiatric Foundation, 1947).
22. Sigmund Freud, The Problem of Anxiety (New York: W. W. Norton & Company, Inc., 1936).
23. Rogers, An Introduction, p. 86.
24. Peplau, Interpersonal Relations, p. 18.
25. Edgar H. Schein, "The Mechanisms of Change," in The Planning of Change, 2nd ed., ed. by Warren G. Bennis and others (New York: Holt, Rinehart & Winston, 1969), p. 99.
26. Peplau, Interpersonal Relations, p. 18.
27. Ibid., p. 30.
28. Ibid., p. 35.
29. Ibid., p. 32.
30. Abraham Maslow, Motivation and Personality (New York: Harper and Row Publishers, Inc., 1954).
31. Hans Selye, The Stress of Life (New York: McGraw-Hill Book Company, 1956).
32. Grayce M. Sills, "Research in the Field of Psychiatric Nursing, 1952-1977." Nursing Research, 26, no. 3 (May-June 1977), 203.
33. Ibid.

7

DOROTHEA E. OREM

Peggy Coldwell Foster and Nancy P. Janssens

Dorothea Orem has been active in both nursing service and nursing education. The positions she has held include Assistant Professor, School of Nursing, The Catholic University of America, Washington, D.C.; Scholar in Residence, School of Nursing, Medical College of Virginia, Richmond, Virginia; and Consultant in Nursing and Nursing Education, Chevy Chase, Maryland.

If you give a man a fish he will have a single meal;
If you teach him how to fish he will eat all his life.
—Kuan-Tzer

Dorothea Orem's concept of nursing, first published in 1959,[1] focuses on the individual.[2] According to Orem, nursing's special concern is: "man's need for self-care action and the provision and management of it on a continuous basis in order to sustain life and health, recover from disease or injury and cope with their effects."[3] Orem further states that "nursing is a way of overcoming human limitations. . . . Nursing developed because man is not self-sufficient."[4]

The following areas in relation to Orem's theory will be discussed:

1. Nursing as a service, an art, and a technology.
2. Premise of self-care.
3. Orem's theory and the nursing process.
4. Orem and the concepts of man, learning, health, society, and nursing.
5. Summary and conclusions.

NURSING AS A SERVICE, AN ART, AND A TECHNOLOGY

Dorothea Orem views nursing as a "community service," an "art," and a "technology." According to Orem, a community is "essentially a group of individuals and families who share not only a common geographic area and environment, but a common interest in the institutions that govern and regulate their way of life."[5]

"Nursing, considered as a health service, is an interpersonal process since it requires the social encounter of a nurse with a patient and involves transaction between them."[6] Nursing, like other services established by the community, must be planned for, maintained, and developed in keeping with the community's needs.[7] "The strength and effectiveness of nursing as a health service in the community depends on the values of that community."[8]

Orem defines the art of nursing as the "ability to assist others in the design, provision and management of systems of self-care to improve or to maintain human functioning at some level of effectiveness."[9] As an art, nursing has an intellectual aspect—the discernment of, and planning for, what can and should be done; and a practical aspect—the giving of care and the overcoming of obstacles to care.[10]

Orem states that the art of nursing needs to include: "(1) the art of helping, (2) the methods of helping, (3) helping techniques appropriate to situations, and (4) nursing systems."[11] All these factors should be included in the education of the beginning nursing student.[12]

Before the nurse can be a helper to an individual, she must be perceived by the person as having the knowledge and the ability to help. There are five different methods of helping or assisting identified in Orem's framework: "(1) acting for or doing for another, (2) guiding another, (3) supporting another, (4) providing an environment that promotes personal development in relation to becoming able to meet present or future demands for action, and, (5) teaching another."[13] Nurses must be aware of these methods of assisting and must select the method that is the most appropriate to the particular situation.[14] The helping aspect of this art is complicated; that is, although the tasks performed may be quite simple, the process of giving and receiving of help to meet a need is affected by the personalities of both the helper and the person needing or perceived to be needing the help.[15]

Orem further identifies nursing as a technology. She states:

> Nursing has formalized methods or techniques of practice, clearly described ways for performing specific actions so that some particular result will be achieved. . . . Techniques of nursing must be learned, and skill and expertness in their use must be developed by persons who pursue nursing as a career.[16]

The types of techniques that nurses use include those concerned with:

> (1) communicating with persons in states of health or disease, (2) bringing about and maintaining interpersonal, intragroup, and intergroup relations for cooperative efforts, (3) giving human assistance adapted to specific human needs and limitations, (4) bringing about, maintaining, and controlling the position and movements of persons in a physical environment for therapeutic purposes, (5) sustaining and maintaining life processes, (6) promoting processes of human growth and development including self or ego development, (7) appraising, changing, and controlling psychophysical modes of human functioning in health and disease, and (8) bringing about and maintaining therapeutic relations based on psychosocial modes of human functioning in health and disease.[17]

She states that although these techniques are used by nurses, they are "not confined to nursing."[18]

PREMISE OF SELF-CARE

According to Orem,

> Self-care is the practice of activities that individuals personally

initiate and perform on their own behalf to maintain life, health, and well-being. . . . It is an *adult's* personal, continuous contribution to his own health and well-being.[19]

It is important to note in Orem's framework that the child is considered to be "a dependent who must be cared for or guided by a responsible adult."[20]

A primary requirement in the practice of self-care is the answer to the questions: Will it benefit me? Can I do it?

Self-care can be described as a deliberate action that is essentially an action to achieve a foreseen result. According to Orem, self-care action is preceded by reflection or judgment to appraise the situation and by a thoughtful deliberate choice of what should be done.[21]

Self-care is a positive action that has both a practical and a therapeutic approach. Self-care may be therapeutic to the extent that it contributes to the achievement of the following elements:

1. Support of life processes and promotion of normal functioning.
2. Maintenance of normal growth, development, and maturation.
3. Prevention, control, or cure of disease processes and injuries.
4. Prevention of, or compensation for, disability.[22]

Self-care is related to many factors: man, environment, culture, and values of daily living.

The concept of *man* would include his internal physical, psychological, and social nature. In contrast, the concept of *environment* would encompass the elements external to man. If one would apply general system theory to Orem's theory, man and environment could be seen to interact as a self-care system. A change in either the system of man or the system of the environment will affect the self-care system. Orem states: "Man's functioning is linked to his environment, and, together, man and environment form an integrated functional whole or system."[23]

Man has adapted his needs to the stresses of the environment; he has utilized technology to control the environment to meet his needs. For example, he has developed various methods to warm his shelter when the environment is cooler than is comfortable.

It would be difficult and probably unsuccessful if the nurse were to implement a needed change without considering how the patient currently meets his daily self-care needs. A failure to consider the patient's environment and life style would most likely prevent the maximal adherence to the new regimen for care.

Self-Care Related to Culture

The way an individual meets his self-care needs is not instinctual, but rather is learned behavior based on one's cultural background.[24] For example, within American society, a patient raised in the Appalachian cultural tradition with a fatalistic approach to health care would probably not seek treatment until his illness prevented him from going to work.[25] The nurse should consider this belief as she attempts to implement preventative health care such as encouraging dental checkups and immunizations.

A person of Spanish culture might support the belief of *mal aire* ("bad air") as a frequent etiology of illness. It is believed that the air may enter the body through any of its openings and may cause disease; hence the practice of the newborn infant wearing a cap to prevent air from entering the ears, and the practice of placing a raisin on the newborn's umbilicus.[26]

The family is the first teacher of the individual's cultural norms. Later in life, other societal units such as friends, teachers, television, and the community impart health care knowledge. Since families, as well as other societal influences, are unique to each individual, many variations of self-care result. Self-care may be an integrated part of the routine *"daily living" activities* requiring minimal attention, or it may be the focus of all activity, such as when an individual has impaired health.[27]

Self-care is not only affected by the individual's position in the family; it is also affected by the person's roles, age, and state of health.[28] A person's value system determines his self-care priorities. For example, a coal miner labors daily in a hazardous occupation to provide a livelihood for his family. To him, obtaining an income for his family is more important than his own health needs.

Kinds of Self-Care

Orem classifies self-care action into two categories: (1) universal self-care and (2) health deviation self-care. *Universal self-care* is defined as all those demands and actions referred to in the literature as

activities of daily living or those that meet basic human needs; and
health deviation self-care is defined as all those demands and actions
that "are required only in the event of illness, injury, or disease."[29]

Universal Self-Care. Orem divides universal self-care demands
and actions into the following six categories: (1) air, water, and food,
(2) excrements, (3) activity and rest, (4) solitude and social interaction,
(5) hazards to life and well-being, and (6) being normal.[30]

Air, water, and food are critical elements for the life processes.
When there is insufficient oxygen to satisfy the normal requirements of
the cells, the individual may experience objective and subjective manifestations that will stimulate him to breathe. To meet therapeutic self-
care needs in regard to air, knowledge of respiration and of the
symptomatology of respiratory dysfunction is required. The sensation
of thirst is caused by fluid and electrolyte variances. To understand the
total mechanism of water metabolism, the nurse must be aware of the
basics of fluid and electrolyte balances. The desire to eat is accom-
panied by a cycle of hunger that is influenced by physiological and
psychological needs and cultural patterns. Therapeutic self-care in this
area necessitates knowledge of nutrition and food metabolism. Normally there is little attention given to the availability of air, water, and
food unless there is a scarcity in quality or quantity.[31]

Excrements are those materials processed or produced by the body
that are no longer of value within the body and are eliminated through
body orifices or directly on the body surface. The normal human
excrements are urine, feces, perspiration, carbon dioxide, menstrual
flow, and seminal fluid. Self-care should include the understanding of
the excretory processes as well as of the social and personal responsibilities regarding them.[32]

A proper balance between *activity and rest* is required for optimal
human functioning. Activity refers to physical, mental, and/or social
actions. Rest connotes a respite from activity, a change from one
activity to another, or the state of sleep.[33]

"Self-care behaviors are the judgments and choices which influence how effort and energy are expended."[34] Therapeutic self-care
requires not only the knowledge and awareness of the physical and
emotional developmental processes, but also the balance between the
two to maintain optimal human functioning. If one has adequate
knowledge and awareness, then valid practical judgments can be
made.[35]

The individual's state of wellness is affected by the conditions of *aloneness and social interactions.* In order for a person to function optimally, there must be a balance between these two areas. However, the quantity and quality of time spent in solitude or in social interactions will vary with each individual's needs. Orem states: "Self-care in this area should be concerned with maintaining that quality and balance of solitary and social experiences necessary for both individual autonomy and enduring social relationships."[36]

There may be *physical, social, and psychological hazards* that affect life and well-being. For example, physical hazards may include acts of nature, accidents, or man-caused changes in the environment; psychological hazards may include dysfunctional coping mechanisms such as substance abuse; and social hazards may include low socioeconomic conditions and lack of recreational facilities. "Self-control and control of environmental conditions are both needed if hazards to life and well-being are to be prevented or controlled."[37]

What is *normal* to one individual or group may not be normal to another. Norms may be guided by three standards in society: (1) the present fad or fashion, (2) scientific criteria for human development (such as those of Erikson or Piaget),[38] and (3) culturally prescribed standards. Self-care related to the "normalcy" concept is comprised of an integrated self-concept, maintenance of the body, and attendance to an impaired health state.[39]

Health Deviation Self-Care.   When the individual cannot meet his own universal self-care needs, he will require health deviation self-care. Orem defines health deviation self-care as that which is "required only in the event of illness, injury, or disease."[40] The actions for such self-care may necessitate adjustment in the following modes:

(1) adjusting the ways of meeting universal self-care requirements; (2) establishing new techniques of self-care; (3) modifying the self-image; (4) revising the routine of daily living; (5) developing a new life-style compatible with the effects of the health deviation; and (6) coping with the effects of the health deviation or the medical care used in the diagnosis or treatment of it.[41]

An illustration of health deviation self-care would be a patient with alterations in elimination (such as a recent colostomy), who would require adjustments in all of the above modes. He would need to adjust his life style to allow for the following: a new means of stool elimination, care for the skin at the colostomy site, a change in his self-image, a revision of activities of daily living to allow time for the colostomy irrigation, an adjustment in his diet to decrease gas formation, and learning to cope with the effects of his illness and its treatment.

Since the nurse is an integral factor in the self-care focus with the patient, it is essential that the nurse recognize the two-facet dimensions of health deviation self-care; that is, that there are demands that arise from the disease itself as well as from the measures that are used in its diagnosis and treatment.[42] It is essential that professional nurses have a knowledge base in pathophysiology and in the supporting sciences to assist the patient in health deviation self-care.

OREM'S THEORY
AND THE NURSING PROCESS

According to Orem, nursing as well as self-care contain both an intellectual and a practical phase. In the nursing process,

> the determination . . . of why a patient requires nursing assistance and her (the nurse's) judgments about how this help can be given [are] essentially intellectual activity. . . . When the nurse begins and continues to perform assisting acts for the patient, nursing is essentially practical activity.[43]

Orem specifically lists the steps of the nursing process as she views it. These steps are included in the intellectual and practical phases. Orem's phases and steps will be compared with the nursing process as defined in Chapter 2 (see Table 7-1).

Orem's Intellectual Phase
(Steps I and II)

In the intellectual phase the nurse must consider the patient's life history and life style. The individual's cultural background affects the usual performance of self-care since this is a learned process.[44]

In the total assessment and data gathering, Orem stresses that the nurse must consider both the medical and the patient's points of view.[45] Thus, the nursing focus must include: the physician's perspective, the patient's perspective, the patient's state of health, the health

Table 7-1

Comparison of Orem's Nursing Process
and the Nursing Process

Orem's Nursing Process	Nursing Process[a]
Intellectual Phase	
Step I—Collect data; determine why a patient needs nursing care; consider patient's life history and life style.	1. Assessment
	2. Diagnosis
Step II—Design of a patient-nursing system; plan for the delivery of nursing care.	3. Planning
Practical Phase	
Step III—Initiate, conduct, and control the actions needed for nursing care.	4. Implementation
Control the delivery of nursing care.	5. Evaluation

[a]Five-step process as outlined in Chapter 2 of this text.

results sought, the patient's requirements for therapeutic self-care, and the present abilities and disabilities of the patient to engage in self-care.[46] *Step I* is "the initial and continuing determination of why a person should be under nursing care"[47] and is part of the intellectual phase. This part when compared with the nursing process of Chapter 2 would be considered as *assessment* and *diagnosis*.

The intellectual phase would also include Orem's Step II of the process. *Step II* is defined as "the designing of a system . . . that will effectively contribute to the patient's achievement of health goals through therapeutic self-care. . . ."[48] Step II also includes the planning for the delivery of nursing care. "The result of Step II should be a mutually agreeable plan. . . ."[49] When compared with the nursing process as defined in Chapter 2, this would include the *planning* of the nursing care.

Orem's Nursing Systems

Orem identifies three basic types of nursing systems to meet the patient's needs for nursing assistance. The design of the system should precede the rendering of assistance by the nurse. According to Orem, the three basic types of nursing systems are: (1) wholly compensatory, (2) partly compensatory, and (3) supportive-educative[50] (see Figure

7-1). "The design of a nursing system is formed by the nurse's selection and use of methods of assisting, since each method prescribes particular roles for the nurse and the patient."[51]

The *wholly compensatory nursing system* is represented by a situation in which the patient has no active role in the performance of care. The nurse "helps" by acting for or doing for the patient. There are three variations in this system: (1) the patient is totally incapacitated, mentally and physically, (2) the patient is in a state of physical incapacitation but is aware of happenings in the environment, and (3) the patient's psychomotor activity is not directed toward meeting requirements for life, safety, or effective human functioning.[52] An example of a person needing care in the wholly compensatory system would be a patient who is nonresponsive. In this situation, the nurse

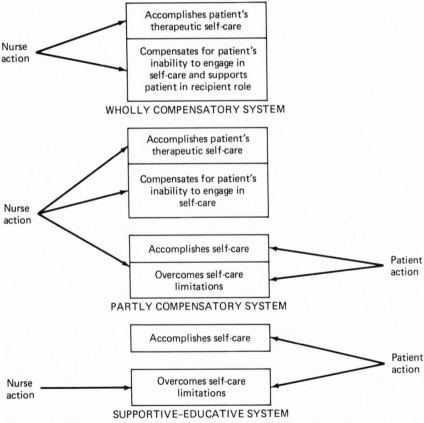

Figure 7-1. Basic nursing systems. [*From* Dorothy E. Orem, *Nursing: Concepts of Practice* (New York: McGraw-Hill Book Company, 1971), p. 78. Used with permission.]

must insure that all of his needs are met, including oxygenation, nutrient intake, elimination, body hygiene, range of motion exercises, and sensory stimulation.

The *partly compensatory nursing system* is represented by a situation in which both the nurse and the patient perform care measures or other actions involving manipulative tasks or ambulation. Either the nurse or the patient may have the major role in the meeting of the needs.[53] An example of a person needing nursing care in the partly compensatory system would be a patient who has had recent surgery. The patient might need much assistance with oral hygiene, toilette, or ambulation. Or the individual might be able to meet most of his self-care needs, and can actively communicate to the nurse the time, the type, and the degree of assistance that is needed.

The *supportive-educative system* is a system where the patient is able, or can and should learn, to perform the required self-care measure, but cannot do so without assitance. The methods of helping or assisting in this system would include: support, guidance, the provision of a developmental environment, and teaching.[54] An example of a person needing care in the supportive-educative system would be an adolescent with a metabolic disorder. When the community health nurse visits the home, the nurse would give support to the patient and his family by listening to their concerns. The nurse would then teach the family the pathophysiology of the impairment, the need for exercise, the technical skills for medication administration, and foot care. The nurse would also guide them in the dietary regime and would encourage them to provide an environment where the adolescent can meet his physical and psychological developmental tasks. This system is discussed by other authors as the supportive-developmental system[55] and is applicable to an individual experiencing a developmental transition, such as middlescence.*

Orem's Practical Phase
(Step III)

Orem's Step III is in essence the practical phase. *Step III is* defined as

---

* "Middlescence or middle adulthood refers to the stages in life when the adult life-style, the occupational mode, and the family life (or single life) pattern have been chosen and the individuals involved settle down to implementing their choices." [Joanne Sabol Stevenson, *Issues and Crises During Middlescence* (New York: Appleton-Century Crofts, 1977), p. 17.]

The initiation, conduction and control of assisting action to (a) compensate for the patient's self-care limitations to insure that self-care is given and is therapeutic and to enable him to adapt his behavior to his limitations, (b) overcome when possible self-care limitations of the patient (or care limitations of the family) so that the patient's future short-term or long-term therapeutic self-care requirements can be met with responsibility, and (c) foster and protect the patient's self-care abilities and prevent the development of new self-care limitations.[56]

When compared with the nursing process as defined in Chapter 2, this would be *implementation.*

Orem speaks about *evaluation* (as defined in Chapter 2) in her Step III of the practical phase when she states that Step III of the nursing process is a cycle of assisting, checking, adjusting, and evaluating activities. "Controlling the delivery of nursing [is] a process of checking what has been done against specification for the actions to be performed."[57]

OREM AND THE CONCEPTS OF MAN, LEARNING, HEALTH, SOCIETY, AND NURSING

It is important when using the nursing process to consider how Orem views the concepts of man, learning, health, society, and nursing.

Orem views *man* as a unity functioning biologically, symbolically, and socially.[58] The individual as the focus for self-care should be considered as an integrated whole. Man and environment form an integrated system.[59] A change in either component may affect the self-care system.

"Education in self-care . . . is necessary for development of knowledge, skills, and positive attitudes related to self-care and health."[60] *Learning* may be a matter of "absorption," such as when a patient observes a competent nurse caring for him. At other times, one may learn from specific and planned learning experiences, such as reading, discussion, and problem solving.[61] This concept is applicable to both the patient in the self-care system and the nurse in Orem's nursing systems.

Health is a state of wholeness or integrity of the individual human being, his parts, and his modes of functioning.[62] This implies that the essence of health is the capacity to live as a human being within one's physical, biologic, and social environment, achieving some measure of the human life potential.[63] This concept is inherent in Orem's nursing systems since the goal in each system is optimal wellness relative to that system. This concept of health acknowledges the patient's integrity and responsibility for his health state.

Orem refers to the concept of *society* when she defines a community as: a body of people living together in the same district, city, or area under the same laws.[64] Societies specify the conditions that make it legitimate for its members to seek various human services necessary to self-care activities.[65] Orem emphasizes that nurses' roles in society focus on the maintenance of self-care.

Nursing's special concern is "man's need for self-care action and the provision and management of it on a continuous basis in order to sustain life and health, recover from disease or injury, and cope with their effects."[66] *Nursing* is a human service based on the values of self-help and help for individuals unable to assist themselves.[67] Orem focuses on the individual as the premise for self-care action.[68] She also describes nursing as the giving of direct assistance to a person, as required, because of the person's specific inabilities in self-care resulting from a situation of personal health.[69] The art of nursing, as defined, is an interpersonal process that includes an intellectual phase and a practical phase.[70] Orem utilizes the nursing process as the basis for professional practice. She states that nursing has "formalized methods or techniques of practice, clearly described ways for performing specific actions so that some particular result will be achieved."[71] This aspect of nursing is inherent in Orem's practical phase of the nursing process and also in the three basic nursing systems.

SUMMARY AND CONCLUSION

A primary strength of Orem's theory of nursing is the incorporation of the major premise of self-care for individuals at various levels of health. Although the family, community, and environment are considered in self-care action, the focus is primarily on the individual. The patient is usually involved in his own self-care. However, a patient who is unaware of happenings or one whose psychomotor functions are not directed toward meeting life requirements or safety would be assigned a position in the wholly compensatory system.[72] This approach seems to imply that if an individual is physically unable to assist with his self-care needs, he cannot participate mentally in his self-care. In both the wholly compensatory and the partly compensatory nursing systems, Orem's focus seems to be on the physical care and to a lesser degree on the psychosocial nursing care of the patient. This approach seems to negate the integration and interaction of the bio-psycho-socio-spiritual aspects of people.

In her three basic nursing systems, Orem conveys the idea that man possesses dynamic potential at differing levels of wellness, but the model representing these systems (see Figure 7-1) seems to require a compartmentalization of individuals, rather than allowing for the infinite variations and fluctuations in an individual's health status. Another strength is in the supportive-educative system. In this system a nurse can intervene with an individual who may be healthy in most regards, but who may be experiencing developmental anxieties and may need support or guidance.

Orem states that the nurse must focus in part on the physician's perspective.[73] The physician is only one member of the health team. It would seem that other perspectives should also be considered (i.e., the family's, the physical therapist's, the nutritionist's, the social worker's, the minister's). Orem refers to the person receiving health care as the "patient." Orem's framework seems to give most of the power for health care to the physician, who is referred to as "he," or "him." In one portion of her book, she states,

> In all nursing situations there is a need for discussion between the patient's nurse(s) and the physician so that the nurse can determine (1) how the physician views the patient's health situation, (2) the health results he seeks for the patient on a day-by-day basis, and (3) the kinds of observations that are relevant from the medical perspective of the physician.[74]

This approach to nursing may be incompatible with the independent, thinking, professional role of the nurse, and reinforces the dependent handmaiden image.

In addition to the premise of self-care, another major strength of Orem's framework is her advocation of the use of the nursing process. She specifically identifies the steps of this process as she views it.

In the dichotomy of the art as having intellectual and practical phases, there is an implication that these two phases are separate and distinct functions. For example, Orem's Step III of the nursing process, which is described as the initiation, conduction, and control of assisting actions, does *not* seem to require intellectual thought but rather is a performance of nursing techniques. This is possibly one weakness in her concept.

Orem's multiple use of terms to classify self-care (e.g., therapeutic, practical, universal, and health deviation) tends to confuse the learner. Confusion may also result from the unclear definition of other concepts. For example, the concept of *system* as used in Orem's nursing systems, is never completely defined and is different than the term *system* of general systems theory and of body systems. Likewise, when she defines nursing as an art, she states that "the art of nursing is concerned with the design, provision, and management of systems of therapeutic self-care,"[75] and at another point, that "the art of nursing is the ability . . . to assist others in the design, provision, and management of systems of self-care."[76] These statements can have very different interpretations. Is the definition of the art of nursing *the design of* or *the assisting of others to do the designing*? It is not clear if therapeutic self-care is only that care given by the nurses that is therapeutic, or if it may also be an act performed by a client or the family that facilitates recovery or development.

Orem's concept of self-care has pragmatic application in nursing practice. Some nursing curricula are based on the premises of self-care, and one independent nursing practitioner uses the concept of self-care as the core of her professional nursing practice.[77]

Orem identifies her framework as "concepts of practice." However, according to the definition of a theory in Chapter 1, this framework may be considered a theory. As such, Orem's framework supports two of the basic characteristics of theories:

1. Theories can interrelate concepts in such a way as to create a different way of looking at a particular phenomenon (i.e., the premise of self-care is incorporated with nursing in the three broad systems of wholly compensatory, partly compensatory, and supportive-educative).

2. Theories contribute to, and assist in, increasing the general body of knowledge within the discipline (i.e., Orem focuses on nursing as a helping art, assisting the individual to meet his self-care needs, as the foundation for nursing practice).

Orem's theory offers a unique way of looking at the phenomenon of nursing. Her work contributes significantly to the development of nursing theories.

NOTES

1. Dorothea E. Orem, *Guides for Developing Curricula for the Education of Practical Nurses* (Washington, D.C.: Government Printing Office, 1959), p. 5.
2. Dorothea E. Orem, *Nursing: Concepts of Practice* (New York: McGraw-Hill Book Company, 1971), p. 48.
3. Ibid., pp. 1–2.
4. Ibid., p. 1.
5. Ibid., p. 53.
6. Ibid., p. 155.
7. Ibid., p. 56.
8. Ibid., p. 57.
9. Ibid., p. 69.
10. Ibid.
11. Ibid.
12. Ibid.
13. Ibid., pp. 70–72.
14. Ibid., p. 73.
15. Ibid., p. 69.
16. Ibid., p. 3.
17. Ibid., p. 4.
18. Ibid., p. 5.
19. Ibid., p. 13.
20. Ibid., p. 130.
21. Ibid., p. 31.
22. Ibid., pp. 19–20.
23. Ibid., p. 14.
24. Ibid.
25. Adina M. Reinhardt and Mildred D. Quinn, *Family-Centered Community Nursing–A Sociocultural Framework* (St. Louis, Mo.: The C. V. Mosby Co., 1973), p. 73.
26. Ibid.
27. Orem, *Nursing: Concepts of Practice*, pp. 15–16.
28. Ibid., p. 16.
29. Ibid., p. 21.
30. Ibid., pp. 21–28.
31. Ibid., p. 21.
32. Ibid., p. 23.
33. Ibid., pp. 23–24.
34. Ibid., p. 24.
35. Ibid., p. 34.
36. Ibid., p. 26.
37. Ibid.

38. Erik Erikson, *Childhood and Society*, 2nd ed. (New York: W. W. Norton & Co., Inc., 1963); Jean Piaget and Bachel Inhelder, *The Psychology of the Child* (New York: Basic Books, 1969).
39. Orem, *Nursing: Concepts of Practice*, pp. 27–28.
40. Ibid., p. 21.
41. Ibid., p. 30.
42. Ibid., pp. 29–30.
43. Ibid., p. 81.
44. Ibid., pp. 83–85.
45. Ibid., p. 49.
46. Ibid., p. 50.
47. Ibid., p. 158.
48. Ibid.
49. Ibid., p. 164.
50. Ibid., pp. 77–80.
51. Ibid., p. 77.
52. Ibid., pp. 78–79.
53. Ibid., pp. 79–80.
54. Ibid., p. 79.
55. The Nursing Development Conference Group, *Concept Formalization in Nursing Process and Product*, 1st ed. (Boston: Little, Brown & Company, 1973), p. 45.
56. Orem, *Nursing: Concepts of Practice*, p. 158.
57. Ibid., p. 172.
58. Ibid., p. 44.
59. Ibid., pp. 13–14.
60. Ibid., p. 44.
61. Ibid., p. 76.
62. Ibid., p. 42.
63. Ibid., p. 43.
64. Ibid., p. 53.
65. Ibid., p. 2.
66. Ibid., pp. 1–2.
67. Ibid., p. 1.
68. Ibid., p. 48.
69. Orem, *Guides for Developing Curricula*, p. 5.
70. Orem, *Nursing: Concepts of Practice*, p. 81.
71. Ibid., p. 3.
72. Ibid., pp. 78–79.
73. Ibid., p. 50.
74. Ibid., p. 160.
75. Ibid., p. 69.
76. Ibid.
77. M. Lucille Kinlein, *Independent Nursing Practice with Clients* (Philadelphia: J. B. Lippincott Co., 1977).

8

FAYE G. ABDELLAH

Suzanne M. Falco

Faye G. Abdellah is the Assistant Surgeon General and Chief Nurse Officer for the U.S. Public Health Services, Department of Health, Education, and Welfare, Washington, D.C. She holds an Ed.D. from Teacher's College, Columbia University, New York, and an LL.D.

In 1960, influenced by the desire to promote client-centered comprehensive nursing care, Abdellah described nursing as a service to individuals, to families, and, therefore, to society. According to Abdellah, nursing is based on an art and science that mold the attitudes, intellectual competencies, and technical skills of the individual nurse into the desire and ability to help people, sick or well, cope with their health needs. It may be carried out under general or specific medical direction. As a comprehensive service, nursing includes:

1. Recognizing the nursing problems of the client.
2. Deciding the appropriate courses of action to take in terms of relevant nursing principles.
3. Providing continuous care of the individual's total health needs.

4. Providing continuous care to relieve pain and discomfort and provide immediate security for the individual.
5. Adjusting the total nursing care plan to meet the client's individual needs.
6. Helping the individual to become more self-directing in attaining or maintaining a healthy state of mind and body.
7. Instructing nursing personnel and family to help the individual do for himself that which he can within his limitations.
8. Helping the individual to adjust to his limitations and emotional problems.
9. Working with allied health professions in planning for optimum health on local, state, national, and international levels.
10. Carrying out continuous evaluation and research to improve nursing techniques and to develop new techniques to meet the health needs of people.[1]

These original premises have undergone an evolutionary process. As a result, in 1973, item 3—"providing continuous care of the individual's total health needs"—was eliminated.[2] Although no reason was given, it can be hypothesized that the words *continuous* and *total* render that service virtually impossible to provide. From these premises, Abdellah's theory was derived.

ABDELLAH'S THEORY

Although Abdellah's writings are not specific as to a theoretical statement, such a statement can be derived by using her three major concepts of health, nursing problems, and problem-solving. Using the definition that a theory states the relationship between concepts, Abdellah's theory would state that nursing is the use of the problem-solving approach with key nursing problems related to the health needs of people. Such a theoretical statement maintains problem-solving as the vehicle for the nursing problems as the client is moved toward health—the outcome.

BASIC CONCEPTS

Health

Although Abdellah never defines it per se, *health* may be defined as the dynamic state of human functioning whereby the individual continually adapts to internal and external stresses in an attempt to achieve maximum potential for daily living.[3] By performing nursing services, the nurse helps the client achieve a state of health. However, in order to effectively perform these services, the nurse must accurately identify the lacks or deficits regarding health that the client is experiencing. These lacks or deficits are the client's health needs.

Nursing Problems

The client's health needs can be viewed as problems. These problems may be *overt* as an apparent condition or *covert* as a hidden or concealed one. Because covert problems can be emotional, sociological, and interpersonal in nature, they are often missed or perceived incorrectly. Yet, in many instances, solving the covert problems may solve the overt problems as well.[4]

Such a view of problems implies a client-centered orientation. Abdellah, however, seems to imply a different viewpoint by her use of nursing problems. She says a *nursing problem* presented by a client is a condition faced by the client or client's family that the nurse through the performance of professional functions can assist them to meet.[5] Abdellah's use of the term *nursing problems* is more consistent with "nursing functions" or "nursing goals." This viewpoint leads to a more nursing-centered orientation.[6]

This nursing-centered orientation to client care seems contrary to the client-centered approach that Abdellah professes to uphold. This apparent contradiction can be explained by her desire to move away from a disease-centered orientation. In her attempt to bring nursing practice into its proper relationship with restorative and preventative measures for meeting total client needs,[7] she seems to swing the pendulum to the opposite pole, from disease orientation to nursing orientation, while leaving the client somewhere in the middle (see Figure 8-1).

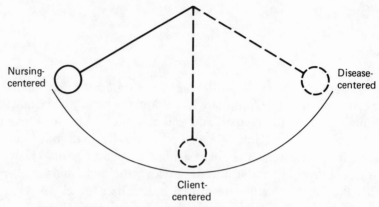

Nursing-
centered

Disease-
centered

Client-
centered

Figure 8-1. The focus of care pendulum.

Problem-Solving

Quality professional nursing care requires that nurses be able to identify and solve overt and covert nursing problems. This can be accomplished by the problem-solving approach. The *problem-solving* process involves identifying the problem, selecting pertinent data, formulating hypotheses, testing hypotheses through the collection of data, and revising hypotheses where necessary on the basis of conclusions obtained from the data.[8]

Many of these steps parallel the steps in the nursing process of assessment, diagnosis, planning, implementation, and evaluation. The problem-solving approach was selected because of the assumption that the correct identification of nursing problems influences the nurse's judgment in selecting the next steps in solving the client's nursing problems.[9] The problem-solving approach is also consistent with such basic elements of nursing practice espoused by Abdellah as observing, reporting, and interpreting the signs and symptoms that comprise the deviations from health and constitute nursing problems; and with analyzing the nursing problems and selecting the necessary course of action.[10]

THE TWENTY-ONE NURSING PROBLEMS

The crucial element within Abdellah's theory is the identification of correct nursing problems. To assist in this identification, the need was defined for a systematic classification of nursing problems presented by

the client. It was felt that such problems could be classified into three
major categories:

1. Physical, sociological, and emotional needs of clients.
2. Types of interpersonal relationships between the nurse and
   client.
3. Common elements of client care.[11]

Over a five-year period, several studies were carried out to establish the classification. As the result of this research, twenty-one groups
of common nursing problems were identified (see Table 8-1). It is
these twenty-one common nursing problems of Abdellah's that are
most widely known, and they will be the focus of the rest of the
chapter.

Table 8-1

The Twenty-One Nursing Problems

1. To maintain good hygiene and physical comfort.
2. To promote optimal activity: exercise, rest, and sleep.
3. To promote safety through the prevention of accidents, injury, or other trauma and
   through the prevention of the spread of infection.
4. To maintain good body mechanics and prevent and correct deformities.
5. To facilitate the maintenance of a supply of oxygen to all body cells.
6. To facilitate the maintenance of nutrition of all body cells.
7. To facilitate the maintenance of elimination.
8. To facilitate the maintenance of fluid and electrolyte balance.
9. To recognize the physiological responses of the body to disease conditions—
   pathological, physiological, and compensatory.
10. To facilitate the maintenance of regulatory mechanisms and functions.
11. To facilitate the maintenance of sensory function.
12. To identify and accept positive and negative expressions, feelings, and reactions.
13. To identify and accept the interrelatedness of emotions and organic illness.
14. To facilitate the maintenance of effective verbal and nonverbal communication.
15. To promote the development of productive interpersonal relationships.
16. To facilitate progress toward achievement of personal spiritual goals.
17. To create and/or maintain a therapeutic environment.
18. To facilitate awareness of self as an individual with varying physical, emotional, and
    developmental needs.
19. To accept the optimum possible goals in the light of limitations, physical and
    emotional.
20. To use community resources as an aid in resolving problems arising from illness.
21. To understand the role of social problems as influencing factors in the cause of
    illness.

Source: From Faye G. Abdellah and others, *Patient-Centered Approaches to Nursing* (New York:
The MacMillan Company, 1960), pp. 16-17. Used with permission.

These twenty-one nursing problems focus on the physical, biological, and social-psychological needs of the client and attempt to
provide a more meaningful basis for organization than the categories of
systems of the body. The most difficult problems were felt to be
numbers 12, 14, 15, 17, 18, and 19.[12] Although a rationale is not
provided for this, it is interesting to note that all these problems fall
into the realm of social-psychological needs and tend to be more
covert in nature.

Within the practice of nursing, it was anticipated that these
twenty-one problems as broad groupings would encourage the generalization of principles and would thereby guide care and promote the
development of the nurse's judgmental ability. Contained in each of
the broad nursing problems are numerous specific overt and covert
problems. It was also anticipated that the constant relating of the broad
basic nursing problems to the specific problems of the individual client
and vice versa would encourage the development of increased ability to
use theory in clinical practice. Thus, a greater understanding of the
relationship between theory and practice would strengthen the usefulness of the nursing problems.[13]

COMPARISON WITH OTHER THEORIES

An examination of these twenty-one problems yields similarities with
other theories. Most notable is their similarity to Henderson's fourteen
components of basic nursing care.[14] As can be seen in Table 8-2,
Abdellah has consolidated some components, such as number 7—
Select suitable clothing, and number 8—Keep body clean and well
groomed; and has expanded others, most notably number 14—Learn,
discover, and satisfy curiosity. The strong similarity may be the result
of both Henderson's and Abdellah's exposure to the same environment—Teacher's College, Columbia University, New York. It might
be hypothesized that Abdellah moved from the rather simplistic form
of Henderson to a more complex structure.

Despite the above similarity, a major difference is evident. Henderson's components are written in terms of client behaviors, whereas
Abdellah's problems are formulated in terms of the nursing services
that should be incorporated into the determination of the client's
needs.[15] This emphasis on nursing services is consistent with Abdellah's apparent nurse-centered orientation mentioned earlier. Hen-

derson seems to have maintained the client-orientation, whereas Abdellah seems to have moved beyond it (see Table 8-2).

Abdellah's nursing problems are also comparable to Maslow's hierarchy of needs.[16] In contrast to Henderson's components, which have a strong physiological orientation, Abdellah's expansion in the *esteem need area* provides a more balanced set of nursing problems between the physical and nonphysical areas (Table 8-2). As with Henderson's components, Abdellah's problems do not meet the self-actualization needs of Maslow. This is not surprising as self-actualization is not a goal to be accomplished, but a process that is ongoing— the dynamic process of becoming. To place elements in this area would negate the dynamism of self-actualization. From a different viewpoint, if Henderson's components and Abdellah's problems are fulfilled, then the client will move toward becoming and self-actualization.

USE OF THE TWENTY-ONE PROBLEMS IN THE NURSING PROCESS

Because of the strong nurse-centered orientation in the twenty-one nursing problems, their use in the nursing process is primarily to direct the nurse. Indirectly, the client benefits. If the nurse helps the client reach all the goals stated in the nursing problems, then the client will be moved toward health.

Within the assessment the nursing problems provide guidelines for the collection of data. A principle underlying the problem-solving approach is that for each identified problem, pertinent data are collected. Thus, for each of the identified twenty-one nursing problems, relevant data are collected. The overt or covert nature of the problems necessitates a direct or indirect approach, respectively. For example, the overt problem of nutritional status can be assessed by direct measures of weight, food intake, and body size; whereas the covert problem of maintaining a therapeutic environment requires more indirect approaches to data collection.

The nursing problems can be divided into those that are basic to all clients and those that reflect sustenal, remedial, or restorative care needs, as seen in Table 8-3. By facilitating data collection, such a classification promotes investigating those problems consistent with the client's stage of illness. However, such a classification promotes the thinking that the client's stage of illness determines appropriate or

Table 8-2

Comparison of Maslow's, Henderson's, and Abdellah's Frameworks

Maslow	Henderson	Abdellah
1. Physiological needs	1. Breathe normally.	5. To facilitate the maintenance of a supply of oxygen to all body cells.
	2. Eat and drink adequately.	6. To facilitate the maintenance of nutrition of all body cells.
		8. To facilitate the maintenance of fluid and electrolyte balance.
	3. Eliminate by all avenues of elimination.	7. To facilitate the maintenance of elimination.
	4. Move & maintain desirable posture.	4. To maintain good body mechanics and prevent and correct deformities.
	5. Sleep & rest.	2. To promote optimal activity: exercise, rest, and sleep.
	6. Select suitable clothing.	10. To facilitate the maintenance of regulatory mechanisms and functions.
	7. Maintain body temperature.	1. To maintain good hygiene and physical comfort.
	8. Keep body clean & well groomed & protect the integument.	
2. Safety needs	9. Avoid environmental dangers & avoid injuring others.	3. To promote safety through the prevention of accident, injury, or other trauma and through the prevention of the spread of infection.
3. Belonging and love needs.	10. Communicate with others.	11. To facilitate the maintenance of sensory function.
		14. To facilitate the maintenance of effective verbal and nonverbal communication.

Maslow	Henderson	Abdellah
		15. To promote the development of productive interpersonal relationships.
		16. To facilitate progress toward achievement of personal spiritual goals.
		19. To accept the optimum possible goals in the light of limitations, physical and emotional.
4. Esteem needs	11. Worship according to faith.	9. To recognize the physiological responses of the body to disease conditions—pathological, physiological, and compensatory.
	12. Work at something providing a sense of accomplishment.	12. To identify and accept positive and negative expressions, feelings, and reactions.
	13. Play or participate in various forms of recreation.	13. To identify and accept the interrelatedness of emotions and organic illness.
	14. Learn, discover, or satisfy curiosity.	17. To create and/or maintain a therapeutic environment.
		18. To facilitate awareness of self as an individual with varying physical, emotional, and developmental needs.
		20. To use community resources as an aid in resolving problems arising from illness.
		21. To understand the role of social problems as influencing factors in the cause of illness.
5. Self-actualization needs		

Table 8-3

The Relationships Among the Classification and Approach of the Twenty-One Nursing Problems and Stages of Illness, Nursing Interventions, and Criterion Measures

Stages of Illness[a]	Nursing Problems	Classification and Approach[b]	Nursing Interventions[c]	Criterion Measures[a]
Basic to all patients	1. To maintain good hygiene and physical comfort. 2. To promote optimal activity: exercise, rest, and sleep. 3. To promote safety through prevention of accident, injury, or other trauma and through the prevention of the spread of infection. 4. To maintain good body mechanics and prevent and correct deformities.	Overt and/or covert problems Direct and/or indirect methods	Measures necessary to maintain hygiene, physical comfort, activity, rest and sleep, safety, and body mechanics.	Related to preventive care needs.
Sustenal care needs	5. To facilitate the maintenance of a supply of oxygen to all body cells. 6. To facilitate the maintenance of nutrition of all body cells. 7. To facilitate the maintenance of elimination. 8. To facilitate the maintenance of fluid and electrolyte balance. 9. To recognize the physiological responses of the body to disease conditions—pathological, physiological, and compensatory. 10. To facilitate the maintenance of regulatory mechanisms and functions. 11. To facilitate the maintenance of sensory function.	Usually overt problems Direct methods	Measures necessary to maintain oxygen supply, nutrition, elimination, fluid and electrolyte balance, regulatory mechanisms, and sensory functions. Interventions imply recognition of body's response to disease.	Related to sustenal and restorative care needs—the normal and disturbed physiological body processes that are vital to sustaining life.

Stages of Illness[a]	Nursing Problems	Classification and Approach[b]	Nursing Interventions[c]	Criterion Measures[a]
Remedial care needs	12. To identify and accept positive and negative expressions, feelings, and reactions. 13. To identify and accept the interrelatedness of emotions and organic illness. 14. To facilitate the maintenance of effective verbal and nonverbal communication. 15. To promote the development of productive interpersonal relationships. 16. To facilitate progress toward achievement of personal and spiritual goals. 17. To create and/or maintain a therapeutic environment. 18. To facilitate awareness of self as an individual with varying physical, emotional, and developmental needs.	Usually covert problems Indirect methods	Measures that are helpful to the client and his family during their emotional reactions to the client's illness.	Related to rehabilitation needs, particularly those involving emotional and interpersonal difficulties.
Restorative care needs	19. To accept the optimum possible goals in the light of limitations, physical and emotional. 20. To use community resources as an aid in resolving problems arising from illness. 21. To understand the role of social problems as influencing factors in the cause of illness.	Overt and/or covert problems Direct and/or indirect methods	Measures that will assist the client and his family to cope with the illness and necessary life adjustment.	Related to sociological and community problems affecting client care.

[a]From Faye G. Abdellah and Eugene Levine, *Better Patient Care Through Nursing Research* (New York: The Macmillan Company, 1965), pp. 78–79, 280–281.

[b]From Faye G. Abdellah and others, *Patient-Centered Approaches to Nursing* (New York: The Macmillan Company, 1973), pp. 81–82.

[c]From Joan Haselman Carter and others, *Standards of Nursing Care* (New York: Springer Publishing Company, 1976), pp. 8–9.

acceptable problems. Such thinking is contrary to the philosophy of holism. If clients are holistic, then they can have needs in any and all areas regardless of the stage of illness. A varied multitude of nursing problems could then exist.

The results of the data collection would determine the client's specific overt and/or covert problems. These specific problems would be grouped under one or more of the broader nursing problems. This step is consistent with that involved in nursing diagnosis. Within this framework, the nursing diagnoses are the exhibited nursing problems.

The twenty-one nursing problems can have a great impact on the planning phase of the nursing process. The statements of the nursing problems most closely resemble goal statements. Therefore, once the problem has been diagnosed, the goals have been established. Many of the nursing-problem statements can be considered goals for either the nurse or the client. Given that these problems are called *nursing problems*, then it becomes reasonable to conclude that these goals are basically *nursing goals*.

Using the goals as the framework, a plan is developed, and appropriate nursing interventions are determined. Table 8-3 summarizes the kinds of interventions that would be appropriate for the categories of nursing problems. Again holism tends to be negated because of the isolated, particulate nature of the nursing problems.

Following implementation of the plan, evaluation takes place. According to the American Nurses' Association *Standards of Nursing Practice*,[17] the plan is evaluated in terms of the client's progress or lack of progress toward the achievement of the stated goals. This would be extremely difficult if not impossible to do for Abdellah's nursing-problem approach, since it has been determined that the goals are *nursing* goals, not *client* goals. Thus, the most appropriate evaluation would be the *nurse's* progress or lack of progress toward the achievement of the stated goals.

Abdellah postulates that criterion measures can be determined from the groupings of the nursing problems, as shown in Table 8-3. A criterion is a value-free name of a measurable variable believed or known to be a relevant indicator of the quality of client care.[18] These criteria can be used to measure client care. Although it is not clear in her writings, the measurement of criteria has been substituted for evaluating a client's progress toward goal achievement.

The use of Abdellah's twenty-one nursing problems in an example might be beneficial. Consider the case of Ron who experiences severe crushing chest pain following a board meeting at his place of business. In addition to the pain, he experiences shortness of breath, tachycardia, and profuse diaphoresis. Upon admission to the hospital, assessment indicates that Ron may have sustained some cardiac damage. Investigation into his history reveals that he has been having episodes of chest pain for the past two months. With this as the data base, the specific problems of pain, impaired cardiac functioning, work-related stress, and failure to seek medical assistance can be identified. These specific problems can be related to selected nursing problems defined by Abdellah, and the nursing problems can be related to the stages of Ron's illness. Nursing strategies and criterion measures can then be determined. Table 8-4 illustrates the implementation of Abdellah's framework. The results of fractionalizing care can be readily seen by the repetition of intervention strategies for the two problems of pain and impaired cardiac functioning. (This table is in no way designed to be inclusive. Rather, it is offered as an attempt to make the theory operational.)

LIMITATIONS

The major limitation to Abdellah's theory and the twenty-one nursing problems is their very strong nursing-centered orientation. With this orientation, appropriate uses might be the organization of teaching content for nursing students and/or the evaluation of student's performance in the clinical area. But in terms of client care, there is little emphasis on what the client is to achieve.

Abdellah's framework is inconsistent with the concept of holism. The classification of the twenty-one nursing problems according to stages of illness and the particulate nature of the problems attest to this. As a result, the client may be diagnosed as having numerous problems, which would lead to fractionalized care efforts, and potential problems might be overlooked because the client is not deemed to be in a particular stage of illness.

CONCLUSIONS

Abdellah's theory and framework provide a basis for determining and organizing nursing care. If all of the problems are investigated, the client would be likely to be thoroughly assessed. The problems also provide a basis for organizing appropriate nursing strategies. It is

Table 8-4

An Illustration of the Implementation of Abdellah's Framework in Ron's Care.

Stages of Illness	Selected Abdellah Nursing Problems	Classification and Approach	Selected Nursing Interventions	Criterion Measures
Basic to care	1. To maintain good hygiene and physical comfort.	Overt problem of pain Direct and indirect methods	1. Administer oxygen. 2. Elevate headrest. 3. Reposition client. 4. Administer prescribed analgesic. 5. Remain with client.	Amount of pain
Sustenal care needs	5. To facilitate the maintenance of a supply of oxygen to all body cells.	Overt problem of impaired cardiac functioning Direct methods	1. Promote rest. 2. Place in sitting position. 3. Promote deep breathing and coughing. 4. Implement exercise program as tolerated.	Vital signs
Remedial care needs	13. To identify and accept the interrelatedness of emotional and organic illness.	Covert problem of effects of work-related stress on cardiac functioning Indirect methods	1. Investigate the nature of his job and activities involved. 2. Explore his work-related goals. 3. Explore the kinds of stress associated with his job.	Knowledge of relationship between stress and his illness
Restorative care needs	20. To use community resources as an aid in resolving problems arising from illness.	Overt problem of failure to seek medical assistance when needed Direct methods	1. Teach early warning signs and symptoms of cardiac distress. 2. Teach course of action should specific symptoms occur.	Knowledge of appropriate use of certain community resources

anticipated that by solving the nursing problems, the client would be moved toward health. The nurse's philosophical frame of reference would determine whether this theory and the twenty-one nursing problems could be implemented in practice.

SUMMARY

Using Abdellah's concepts of health, nursing problems, and problem-solving, the theoretical statement of nursing that can be derived is the use of the problem-solving approach with key nursing problems related to the health needs of people. From this framework, twenty-one nursing problems were developed. These problems are compared to Henderson's fourteen components of nursing and Maslow's hierarchy of needs. Ways to utilize the nursing problems in the nursing process are explored. The major limitation of Abdellah's theory is its strong nursing-centered orientation. Some modification of the nursing problems to promote a more client-centered orientation would encourage effective utilization of the theory in professional nursing practice.

NOTES

1. Faye G. Abdellah and others, *Patient-Centered Approaches to Nursing* (New York: The Macmillan Company, 1960), pp. 24–25.
2. Faye G. Abdellah and others, *New Directions in Patient-Centered Nursing* (New York: The Macmillan Company, 1973), p. 19.
3. Wright State University School of Nursing, *Glossary of Terms* (Dayton, Ohio: Wright State University School of Nursing, 1975).
4. Abdellah and others, *Patient-Centered Approaches*, pp. 6–7.
5. Ibid.
6. Marion E. Nicholls and Virginia G. Wessells, eds., *Nursing Standards and Nursing Process* (Wakefield, Mass.: Contemporary Publishing, Inc., 1977), p. 6.
7. Abdellah and others, *Patient-Centered Approaches*, pp. 30–31.
8. Ibid., pp. 6, 26.
9. Faye G. Abdellah and Eugene Levine, *Better Patient Care Through Nursing Research* (New York: The Macmillan Company, 1965), p. 492.
10. Abdellah and others, *Patient-Centered Approaches*, p. 26.
11. Ibid., p. 11.
12. Abdellah and others, *New Directions*, p. 79.
13. Abdellah and others, *Patient-Centered Approaches*, p. 27.

14. Virginia Henderson and Gladys Nite, *Principles and Practice of Nursing*, 6th ed. (New York: The Macmillan Company, 1978), p. 94.
15. Lillian DeYoung, *The Foundations of Nursing* (St. Louis, Mo.: The C. V. Mosby Co., 1976), p. 112.
16. Abraham Maslow, *Motivation and Personality* (New York: Harper and Row Publishers, Inc., 1954).
17. Congress for Nursing Practice, *Standards of Nursing Practice* (Kansas City, Mo.: American Nurses' Association, 1973).
18. Doris Bloch, "Criteria, Standards, Norms—Crucial Terms in Quality Assurance," *Journal of Nursing Administration*, 7, no. 1 (September 1977, 22.

REFERENCES

ABDELLAH, FAYE G., and others, *New Directions in Patient-Centered Nursing*. New York: The Macmillan Company, 1973.

———*Patient-Centered Approaches to Nursing*. New York: The Macmillan Company, 1960.

——— and EUGENE LEVINE, *Better Patient Care Through Nursing Research*. New York: The Macmillan Company, 1965.

BLOCH, DORIS, "Criteria, Standards, Norms—Crucial Terms in Quality Assurance," *Journal of Nursing Administration*, 7, no. 1 (September 1977), 20–30.

BYRNE, MARJORIE L., and LIDA F. THOMPSON, *Key Concepts for the Study and Practice of Nursing*. St. Louis, Mo.: The C. V. Mosby Co., 1972.

CARTER, JOAN HASELMAN, and others, *Standards of Nursing Care*. New York: Springer Publishing Company, Inc., 1976.

CONGRESS FOR NURSING PRACTICE, *Standards of Nursing Practice*. Kansas City, Mo.: American Nurses' Association, 1973.

DEYOUNG, LILLIAN, *The Foundations of Nursing*. St. Louis, Mo.: The C. V. Mosby Co., 1976.

HENDERSON, VIRGINIA, and GLADYS NITE, *Principles and Practice of Nursing*, 6th ed. New York: The Macmillan Company, 1978.

NICHOLLS, MARION E., and VIRGINIA G. WESSELS, eds. *Nursing Standards and Nursing Process*. Wakefield, Mass.: Contemporary Publishing, Inc., 1977.

WRIGHT STATE UNIVERSITY SCHOOL OF NURSING, *Glossary of Terms*. Dayton, Ohio: Wright State University School of Nursing, 1975.

9

IDA JEAN ORLANDO

Mary Disbrow Crane

At the time The Dynamic Nurse-Patient Relationship *was pub-lished,*[1] *Ida Jean Orlando was Associate Professor of Mental Health and Psychiatric Nursing and Director of the Graduate Program in Mental Health and Psychiatric Nursing at Yale University School of Nursing. Her highest degree achieved was a Master of Arts. The book was an outgrowth of a five-year project that began in 1954 under a National Institute of Mental Health Grant.*

Another significant contributor to the developing body of nursing theory is Ida Jean Orlando. Orlando's theory describes a nursing process based on the interaction taking place in a specific time and place between a patient and a nurse. Her purpose was to produce a "theory of effective nursing practice."[2] She attempted the integration of function, process, and principles to describe the uniqueness of the role of the professional nurse.

As with the development of all other theories, some understanding of Orlando's background and the times in which the theory was developed will provide insight into her work. Orlando's advanced nursing preparation and her position in the educational setting were in the area of mental health and psychiatric nursing. Her theory was developed in the middle to late 1950s during a project that sought to identify factors affecting the integration of mental health principles into basic nursing curricula. This study involved extensive observation of nurse-patient interactions utilizing nurses at various points in their professional preparation and in various practice settings. The concerns facing nursing at that time, to which Orlando wished to contribute, were: "nurse-patient relationships, the nurse's professional role and identity, and the development of knowledge which is distinctly nursing."[3]

KEY CONCEPTS

Certain major concepts are critical to Orlando's theory of nursing. She views that which is *unique* to nursing as the *process* involved in *interacting* with an *ill individual* to meet an *immediate need*. This interaction is *dynamic* because the situation is constantly changing. An initial focus on each of these concepts (uniqueness, process, interaction, individual, immediate need, dynamic) will provide a basis for examining her nursing process.

Orlando was concerned with what was *uniquely nursing*. Therefore, she developed a theory that can be applied with equal ease to any of the specialty areas into which nursing has been traditionally divided. Her focus on understanding what is happening between patient and nurse makes her theory equally applicable to nursing children, surgical patients, or patients with mental health problems. Orlando defines the nursing function as "the direct responsibility to see to it that the patient's needs for help are met either by her [the nurse's] own action or by calling in the help of others."[4] This nursing function is differentiated from that of medicine, to which Orlando attributes responsibility for the prevention and treatment of disease. Nursing is oriented to the patient, whereas medicine focuses on the disease.

Orlando's theory discusses the uniqueness of nursing from a *process*, rather than from a function, orientation. The nurse is defined by the process of interaction with the patient rather than by the activities she carries out.* Thus, the nurse ascertains the patient's needs, determines appropriate actions to meet them, and sees that

---

*In this chapter, the feminine pronoun is used when referring to the nurse. Although men have entered the nursing profession, they had not done so in significant numbers when Orlando wrote her book. The term *patient* is also used exclusively in place of *client*, as Orlando refers only to individuals who are ill.

these actions are implemented. She may carry out the actions herself or direct auxiliary personnel to do so. Although knowledge of general principles from other disciplines is seen as useful, it is not crucial as long as the patient's need is met either by the nurse or by appropriate referral. What is of sole importance is an effective nurse-patient relationship culminating in a resolved patient need.

If Orlando's theory can be described in any one term, it would be *interactive*. In her own words, "Learning how to understand what is happening between herself and the patient is the central core of the nurse's practice and comprises the basic framework for the help she gives to patients."[5]

Her nursing process is the interaction of the following elements with each other: "the behavior of the patient, the reaction of the nurse, and the nursing actions which are designed for the patient's benefit."[6] These elements form the basis for nursing principles. Nursing practice, then, according to Orlando, begins with and is based on the establishment by the nurse of a helping relationship with the patient.

Because of the interactive nature of Orlando's theory, the *individual* receives prime consideration. Open communication with the patient is essential. The entire nursing process involves the nurse sharing her reactions with the patient to explore the meaning of her/his behavior, the exact nature of the need, what nursing action is appropriate to meet this need, and whether the action was helpful. Thus, the course for the nurse to take with two patients presenting the same behavior (as perceived by the nurse) would differ since patients are individuals with their own manner of expressing needs and responsiveness to a specific action. Cognizance of Orlando's concept of patient individuality can help the nurse to avoid ineffectiveness in her practice due to overgeneralization from one patient to another.

In Orlando's estimation, no nursing care is necessary unless patients perceive a need that they cannot meet by themselves. She defines *need* situationally as "a requirement of the patient which, if supplied, relieves or diminishes immediate distress or improves the immediate sense of well-being."[7] Thus, not all ill persons require nursing care. The nurse is called upon if the patient "cannot deal with what he needs" or "cannot carry out the (medically) prescribed treatment or diagnostic plan alone."[8] Although the patient may have difficulty in communicating the need, it is the patient who determines this need. The nurse's responsibility is to be certain she has correctly identified the need as the patient experiences it.

This need orientation is supported by the *illness* focus of Orlando's theory. Nurses work only with ill persons and access to nursing care comes only through a physician who identifies the illness. The physician is in charge of the patient's care. In Orlando's estimation, nursing offers help to the patient "for his physical and mental comfort to be assured as far as possible while he is undergoing some form of medical treatment or supervision."[9]

Last of all, Orlando's theory focuses on the *immediate* situation. Thus her concept is *dynamic* because situation, time, and place change. Need is defined in terms of the present. Applied to practice, this prevents the nurse from assuming that an intervention that was effective in a previous similar occasion will automatically be appropriate in the current situation. Data must first be collected to determine the usefulness of the action at this time. These concepts are consistent with Martha Rogers's principle of synchrony, which states, "Change in the human field depends upon the state of the human field and the simultaneous state of the environmental field at any given point in space-time."[10]

ORLANDO'S NURSING PROCESS

A more detailed review of Orlando's nursing process is now possible with these major concepts in mind. In her work, the terms *nursing situation* and *nursing process* are used interchangeably. To avoid confusion, *nursing situation* will be used here in discussing Orlando's theory, and *nursing process* will refer to the activity described in Chapter 2 of this book. Orlando's nursing situation is composed of three elements: (1) patient behavior, (2) the nurse's reaction, and (3) nursing actions appropriate to the patient's need. Further elaboration on her use of needs and observation will form the basis for the analysis of these elements.

According to Orlando, when a patient experiences a need that he cannot resolve, distress occurs. Unmet needs that require nursing assistance generally fall into three categories: "physical limitations, adverse reactions to the setting or experiences which prevent the patient from effectively communicating his needs."[11] Distress due to physical limitations may result from incomplete development, temporary or permanent disability, or restrictions of the environment, real or imagined. Adverse reactions to the setting, on the other hand, usually result from incorrect or inadequate understanding of an experience there. Patients may experience distress from an adverse reaction to any aspect of the environment despite its helpful or therapeutic intent. Frequently distress may also result from patients' inability to effectively communicate their needs. This may be due to many factors such as ambivalence concerning the dependency brought on by illness, embarrassment related to the need, lack of trust in the helping person, or inability to state the need effectively. The patient's inability to effectively communicate his needs points to two aspects of the nurse's function:

> First the nurse must take the initiative in helping the patient express the specific meaning of his behavior in order to ascertain his distress. Second, she must help the patient explore the distress in order to ascertain the help he requires for his need to be met.[12]

Observation forms the factual basis for the effective determination and resolution of patient needs. It is defined by Orlando as "any information pertaining to the patient which the nurse acquires while she is on duty."[13] Indirect data are received from any sources other than the patient, such as from records, other health team members, or the patient's family and friends. Direct data are comprised of "any perception, thought or feeling the nurse has from her own experience of the patient's behavior at any or several moments in time."[14] Both types of nursing data require sufficient exploration with patients in order to determine relevance to the specific situation. Orlando offers the following principle to guide the nurse in her collection of nursing data: "Any observation shared and explored with the patient is immediately useful in ascertaining and meeting his need or finding out that he is not in need at that time."[15]

Patient's Behavior

The nursing situation is initiated by a patient behavior. The importance that the nurse should give to any patient behavior is stressed by the following principle: "The presenting behavior of the patient, regardless of the form in which it appears, may represent a plea for help."[16] Thus all patient behavior, no matter how insignificant it may appear to be in the nurse's perception, must be considered an expression of need until its meaning to that particular patient at that time is understood. Patient behavior may be verbal or nonverbal. Verbal behavior encompasses all the nurse hears the patient say. Such behavior may take the form of "complaints, requests, questions, re-fusals, demands and comments or statements."[17] Nonverbal behavior may be perceived by the nurse visually in the case of physiological manifestations and motor activity or through hearing of vocal patient behavior such as crying, laughing, or sighing. Verbal and nonverbal behaviors correspond roughly with subjective and objective data col-lected in the assessment phase of the nursing process. Patient behavior initiates the nursing situation and assessment begins the nursing proc-ess. Both verbal and nonverbal behaviors are useful throughout in validation of the precise nature of the patient needs and of the effectiveness and appropriateness of nursing actions to meet these needs.

Patient behavior, however, is not always helpful. Ineffective be-havior may lead to problems in the nurse-patient relationship. Such behavior "prevents the nurse from carrying out her concerns for the patient's care or from maintaining a satisfactory relationship to the patient."[18] Although behaviors that seem unreasonable, uncooperative, or demanding may provoke negative feelings in the nurse, recognition that they express the distress of the patient can help to control these feelings. Ineffective patient behavior may indicate difficulties in the initial establishment of the nurse-patient relationship, inaccurate ascer-tainment of the patient's need by the nurse, or negative patient reac-tion to automatic nursing actions inappropriate to relieve the patient's distress. Resolution of ineffective patient behavior deserves high pri-ority as the behavior usually increases over time if the need it expresses remains unmet.

Nurse's Reaction

Any patient behavior, or occasionally the nurse's observation of the patient's environment, provokes the next step in the nursing situa-tion—reaction of the nurse. The professional nurse learns to explore her personal reactions for their professional reference and validity. An undisciplined reaction involves almost simultaneous perception of the patient's behavior, automatic thoughts based on this perception, and with the assumption of the correctness of these thoughts, a certain feeling.[19] These reactions may be influenced by the nurse's personal value system or code of behavior or by unresolved reactions to other persons or to constraints of the environment. For example, a nurse may become angry because she believes a patient should not behave in a demanding manner, or she may not respond appropriately to the patient's behavior because of supervisory pressure to carry out a routine task. Such reactions refer to the individual nurse or the environment but have little or nothing to do with the particular patient. Through learning, the nurse develops a responsive discipline that changes the automatic nature of her perceptions, thoughts, and feelings into a process questioning their meaning to the patient. This process leads her to share her perceptions, thoughts, or feelings with patients in a manner that will invite them to respond as to the validity of these perceptions, thoughts, and feelings. This process also requires that reactions to other persons and to the environment be constructively resolved through exploration, so the patient's needs may be the nurse's sole concern. In this area, Orlando's belief in the responsibility and accountability of the nurse is strongly expressed. She states that the nurse is "responsible to resolve extraneous reactions, positive or negative, which interfere with helping patients."[20]

As a result of this discussion, it becomes clear that the nurse's perceptions, thoughts, or feelings are not as important as whether she effectively explores their validity with the patient. Which of the three parts of her reaction (perceptions, thoughts, feelings) she chooses to share with patients is usually not critical as long as she does so in a manner inviting an honest response. In situations requiring immediate action, sharing a perception may lead to quicker clarification than would the statement of a thought resulting from this perception. For example, there is less assumption in the statement, "You are grimacing" than in the question "Are you in pain?" Orlando states that "the patient can make use of the nurse's feeling when [the nurse] expresses it, provided [the nurse] explains the basis for it and allows the patient to correct or validate what [the nurse's] feeling is about."[21] Feelings not openly shared with the patient are usually expressed through nonverbal behavior, which the patients must interpret in their own way and which may not be correct or helpful to their care. Orlando's emphasis on open sharing of the nurse's reaction with the patient provides a sound basis for effective nursing practice. She offers this sharing in the form of a principle to guide the nurse in her reaction to patient behavior: "The nurse does not assume that any aspect of her reaction to the patient is correct, helpful, or appropriate until she checks the validity of it in exploration with the patient."[22]

The nurse's reaction can be compared to the analysis in the assessment phase of the nursing process (see Figure 9-1). Both are deliberate, intellectual attempts to examine the data collected to correctly identify the patient's problem. Total reliance on intuition or feelings is inappropriate. The nursing process stresses the use of a

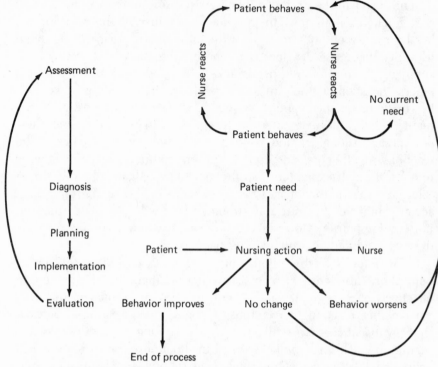

Figure 9-1. Comparison of the nursing process and Orlando's nursing situation.

theoretical and scientific base in analysis, whereas the nursing situation examines the nurse's perceptions, thoughts, and feelings in a more personal manner. If the data have been adequately and accurately collected, the nurse's reaction results in her correct identification of the patient's need as he perceives it, and the analysis leads to the nursing diagnosis.

Nurse's Actions

Once the nurse has validated or corrected her reaction to the patient's behavior through exploration of it with him, she can carry out the final part of the nursing situation, the nurse's actions. Orlando includes "only what she (the nurse) says or does with or for the benefit of the patient"[23] as part of a nurse's actions.

There are two types of nursing actions: (1) automatic and (2) deliberative. Automatic actions are "those decided upon for reasons other than the patient's immediate need," whereas deliberative actions ascertain or meet this need.[24] There is a distinction here between the purpose an action actually serves and its intention to help the patient. For example, a nurse may administer a sleeping pill because the doctor ordered it. Here carrying out the doctor's order is the action's purpose. If, however, the nurse has not determined that the patient is having trouble sleeping or that the pill is the most appropriate method for meeting the need for help in sleeping, the action is not helping the patient. The action is automatic, not deliberative.

Thus, it can be seen that the following conditions differentiate automatic actions from deliberative ones. First, deliberative actions result from patients' needs correctly ascertained after validation of the nurse's reaction to patient behavior. Second, the meaning of the action to patients and its relevance to meeting their needs is explored in deliberative nursing before an action is carried out or a request refused. Next, the effectiveness of the action on resolving the need is explored with the patients immediately after its completion. Finally, deliberative actions are carried out by a nurse free of stimuli unrelated to patients' needs. Automatic actions are more likely to be done by nurses primarily concerned with a doctor's orders, routines of patient care, or principles involved in protecting the health of people in general, and by nurses who do not validate their reactions to patient behavior.

The nurse's action relates to the planning and implementation phases of the nursing process (see Figure 9-1). Both Orlando's situation and the nursing process mandate participation of the patient in planning the care.[25] The nursing process is more comprehensive in requiring written goals and prioritized plans directed toward the resolution of the nursing diagnosis. In the nursing action, planning involves determining, based on the patient's perception, the appropriate action to meet the need. Implementation and the nurse's action are both actions involved in carrying out what is planned.

Inherent in Orlando's theory, as well as in the nursing process, is the necessity for evaluation of the effectiveness of the nurse's actions (see Figure 9-1). For actions to be deliberative, the patient should be consulted for the appropriateness of an action before it is carried out and for its effectiveness after it is completed. Failure to do this may result in a series of ineffective actions with a delay in the patient's improvement and an increase in the cost of nursing care and materials. The success of a nursing action is measured by a change in the patient's behavior. Consistency between verbal and nonverbal behavior is necessary to confirm this evaluation. Thus, according to Orlando, nursing effectiveness must be measured in terms of patient outcomes rather than by what the nurse does, and if the action proves ineffective, a new one is decided on. This part of Orlando's theory was perhaps ahead of her time. In an American Nurses' Association publication, outcomes are described as "the ultimate indicators of quality patient care."[26] To emphasize the importance of evaluating the nurse's actions, the principle guiding nursing activity states, "The nurse initiates a process of exploration to ascertain how the patient is affected by what she says or does."[27]

It is also inherent in this theory that the setting and the nurse's functions both be structured to ensure the nurse maximum freedom to meet the patient's need. Actions appropriate to the patient's need must take precedence over a doctor's order, and the nurse must be free and must accept the responsibility to resolve the conflict. Orlando writes, "Her use of the (medical) order would necessarily take into consideration the responsiblity inherent in any act a nurse performs with or for the patient; i.e., it would consider how the activity affects the patient."[28] Routines of care must be reduced to an absolute minimum, allowing room for the individuality of patients' needs. Since "a nurse's activity is professional only when it deliberately achieves the purpose of helping the patient,"[29] nonprofessional routine activities should be carried out as much as possible by nonnursing personnel. Finally, elements of the setting should minimize the nurse's concern with general protective measures for patients and should avoid stimuli detracting from the nurse's focusing on the patient's need. This is not to deny the necessity of deciding on certain automatic actions needed in the nursing situation, such as certain routines of care and protection of patient safety and of the organization. When this must occur, the nurse can recognize these actions as automatic and can evaluate their effect on the patient before or after the particular action is taken. Actions can then be taken to resolve any conflict between the automatic action and the patient's need, making the process as deliberative as possible.

STRENGTHS AND LIMITATIONS

Orlando's theory is useful in guiding the nurse in her interaction with a patient who is aware of what he needs in a specific time and place. Her theory does, however, have some significant limitations, limitations that can largely be remedied in the nursing process. Since the patient identifies the need, the theory does not apply to situations where the patient may be unaware or unmotivated in an area affecting his health or where he is functioning at a low level of consciousness. A statement of the need is incongruent with problem-solving theory as the solution is reached without a statement of the problem. Individuals only may be viewed as the patient, rather than a family or a community. Orlando also views nursing care as only related to ill persons and provides for no access to nursing care except through a physician. Long-term planning with goals as found in the nursing process has no place in Orlando's theory. She recognizes this deficit and suggests that long-term benefits may be derived from the cumulative effect of being helped in many individual situations.[30] Assessment is also limited to the immediate situation, which restricts the observation of patterns of behavior and accumulation of data to support a conclusion.

Nevertheless, Orlando does provide much guidance in applying the nursing process to patients. Her theory reinforces nursing as a deliberate intellectual activity. It would be impossible with Orlando's theory to exclude the patient from active involvement in any part of the nursing process. Her theory also helps prevent false assumptions leading to an inaccurate diagnosis or inappropriate plan because validation is constantly required. In nursing practice, her theory focuses attention on the patient's needs rather than on those of the health care system because this focus is required for any activity to be professional. Any nurse applying Orlando's theory would have difficulty forgetting to evaluate patient care.

Ida Jean Orlando can be considered a nursing theorist who made significant contributions to nursing practice and its advancement. She helped to switch nursing's focus from the institution or the disease to the patient. She advocated the nurse as a handmaiden of the patient rather than of the physician. She helped make nurses leaders and logical thinkers in their practices rather than followers acting solely on orders or on intuition. Her nursing process continues to be useful as a guide for the nurse's interaction with a particular patient at a given place in time.

ORLANDO AS A NURSING THEORIST

Yet, based on the criteria in Chapter 1 of this book, can Orlando's work be called a theory? Does it relate concepts to develop significant interrelationships to describe or classify approaches to practice?* To

*See Chapter 1, pp. 4-5.

answer these questions a review of Orlando's work relative to the characteristics of a theory is necessary.

The first question to be resolved is Orlando's use of principles to guide nurses in their practice. Principles, as stated in Chapter 1, are useful to pure sciences. They are useful in areas of study where an outcome can be accurately predicted for a given set of circumstances. Human beings, however, are highly individualistic, as Orlando recognizes, and this makes precise prediction difficult. Orlando's principles are general enough to guide practice but actually speak little of outcome. They state how the nurse should act but not what behavior can be expected from the patient. Thus, they might be more appropriately called *guides* for practice rather than actual principles.

The first characteristic of a theory involves the interrelation of concepts to provide a different way of viewing a phenomenon. Nursing usually includes the concepts of humanity, society, health, and nursing in its theoretical base. Orlando uses this concept of humanity with a heavy emphasis on individuality and changeability in relation to time and place. Her concept related to health is mainly a concept of ill-health, because nursing for her is only involved on the illness side of the health continuum. Society as a concept is largely ignored in her work, which deals with the interaction between a specific nurse and a specific patient at a particular time. By combining these concepts with nursing, Orlando is saying that nursing interacts with humanity to alleviate a need related to illness that an individual human being cannot alone resolve. Thus, Orlando does relate concepts into a new and meaningful whole.

Is Orlando's theory logical in nature? It does provide a reasonable and sequential process for nursing. Patient behavior initiates a nurse reaction that helps to determine a nursing activity appropriate to resolve the need that the initial behavior expressed. Orlando places heavy emphasis on careful analysis of each aspect of the process. The nurse's reaction must be controlled to assure accurate identification of the patient's need. The appropriateness of the nursing activity to meet this need must be validated before and after its completion. Thus, Orlando provides nursing with a logical rather than intuitive approach to practice.

Orlando's principles also provide a mechanism for testing. Is there similarity in outcome when the nurse behaves as directed by her principles? Does this similarity occur in a variety of nursing situations? Orlando wished to develop a theory useful to nursing as a whole. Application of her principles in various nursing settings could help to measure her success. The problem lies in the broad generality of her principles, which makes specific testing difficult.

Orlando can definitely be credited with adding to the general body of nursing knowledge. Her general emphasis was extremely helpful in her search for what is uniquely nursing, her insistence on the nurse's accountability to the patient, and her focus of all professional nursing activities on the client. She has minutely dissected the interaction between patient and nurse through observation of hundreds of such occurrences and has provided a framework to guide the course of such interaction. The influence of, or at least consistency with, her theory is certainly evident in the nursing process as it has evolved and in the later work of nursing theorists such as Orem.*

Orlando has succeeded in her efforts to create a theory useful to practice. Nurses can use her principles to guide their interaction with a patient. With the help of these principles, nursing practice is directed so nurses act on the basis of a sound data base rather than on intuition. Her theory is much more easily applied to practice than that of other nursing thinkers of her time. For example, Abdellah's twenty-one problems, developed from an educational framework, lend themselves more easily to the educational than the practice setting. Orlando's theory, however, does not help with certain aspects of nursing such as long-term planning, dealing with family and community, and motivating patients toward improved health practices when no need is perceived by the patient.

Orlando's theory does not directly conflict with other validated theories if it is viewed as dealing with the aspect of nursing that involves a situational encounter between a patient and a nurse revolving around a need. It is most consistent with interactive theory. However, difficulties arise when relating Orlando's theory to systems theory. Although she does recognize that extraneous input from the system interferes with effective nurse reaction, she does not discuss how various suprasystems affect patient behavior and perception of need. For this same reason, it is difficult to relate her theory to family theory. The family is seen only as a source of indirect data.

SUMMARY

For Orlando the nursing situation is rooted in the interaction between a nurse and a patient at a specific time and place. A sequence of interchanges involving patient behavior and nurse reaction takes place

*See Chapter 7, pp. 90-106.

until the patient's need, as perceived by the patient, is clarified. The nurse, then, in cooperation with the patient, decides on an appropriate action to alleviate the need and sees that this activity is carried out. Finally, evaluation of whether or not the need has been met is carried out based on change in the patient's presenting behavior. If the behavior improves, the process ends. If there is no change or if the condition deteriorates, the process recycles with new efforts to clarify the presenting behavior or the appropriateness of the nursing activity (see Figure 9-1). Thus, in Orlando's words,

> A deliberate nursing process has elements of continuous reflection as the nurse tries to understand the meaning to the patient of the behavior she observes and what he needs from her in order to be helped. Responses comprising this process are stimulated by the nurse's unfolding awareness of the particulars of the individual situation.[31]

NOTES

1. Ida Jean Orlando, *The Dynamic Nurse-Patient Relationship: Function, Process and Principles* (New York: G. P. Putnam's Sons, 1961).
2. Ibid., p. viii.
3. Ibid.
4. Ibid., p. 22.
5. Ibid., p. 4.
6. Ibid., p. 36.
7. Ibid., p. 5.
8. Ibid. (parentheses added).
9. Ibid.
10. Martha E. Rogers, *An Introduction to the Theoretical Basis of Nursing* (Philadelphia: F. A. Davis Company, 1970), p. 98.
11. Orlando, *The Dynamic Nurse-Patient Relationship*, p. 11.
12. Ibid., p. 26.
13. Ibid., p. 31.
14. Ibid., p. 32.
15. Ibid., pp. 35–36.
16. Ibid., p. 40.
17. Ibid., p. 37.
18. Ibid., p. 78.
19. Ibid., p. 48.
20. Ibid., p. 60.
21. Ibid., p. 49.

22. Ibid., p. 56.
23. Ibid., p. 60.
24. Ibid.
25. Congress of Nursing Practice, *Standards of Nursing Practice* (Kansas City, Mo.: American Nurses' Association, 1973).
26. Congress of Nursing Practice, A *Plan for Implementation of the Standards of Nursing Practice* (Kansas City, Mo.: American Nurses' Association, 1975), p. 16.
27. Orlando, *The Dynamic Nurse-Patient Relationship*, p. 67.
28. Ibid., p. 77.
29. Ibid., p. 70.
30. Ibid., p. 90.
31. Orlando, *The Dynamic Nurse-Patient Relationship*, p. 67.

10

ERNESTINE WIEDENBACH

Agnes M. Bennett and Peggy Coldwell Foster

Ernestine Wiedenbach, a graduate of Wellesley College, Wellesley, Massachusetts, received her diploma from the Johns Hopkins School of Nursing, Baltimore, Maryland. Her Master's degree is from Teachers College, Columbia University in New York. She obtained a certificate in nurse midwifery from the Maternity Center Association in New York. She has practiced as a nurse midwife and a public health nurse and has taught in a number of schools of nursing. She is an Associate Professor Emeritus from Yale University School of Nursing.

According to Ernestine Wiedenbach, nursing is nurturing and caring for someone in a motherly fashion. That care is given in the immediate present, and can be given by any caring person.[1] Nursing is a helping service that is rendered with compassion, skill, and understanding to those in need of care, counsel, and confidence in the area of health.[2] The practice of nursing comprises a wide variety of services, each directed toward the attainment of one of its three components: (1) identification of the patient's need for help, (2) ministration of the help needed, and (3) validation that the help provided was indeed helpful to the patient.[3]

Wiedenbach states that the characteristics of a professional person that are essential for the professional nurse include: (1) *clarity* of purpose, (2) *mastery* of skills and knowledge essential for fulfilling her purpose,* (3) *ability* to establish and sustain purposeful working relationships with others in the health care field, (4) *interest* in advancing knowledge in her area of interest and in researching new knowledge, and (5) *dedication* to furthering the good of man.[4]

WIEDENBACH'S PRESCRIPTIVE THEORY

After her work with J. Dickoff and P. James in the late 1960s in which they presented a symposium on "Theory in a Practice Discipline,"[5] Wiedenbach wrote *Meeting the Realities in Clinical Teaching.*[6] It was at this time that she began to develop her theory of nursing.

A prescriptive theory (a situation-producing theory) is one that conceptualizes both the desired situation and the prescription used to bring about that desired situation. Wiedenbach's prescriptive theory is made up of three factors:

1. The *central purpose,* which the practitioner recognizes as essential to the particular discipline.
2. The *prescription* for the fulfillment of the central purpose.
3. The *realities in the immediate situation* that influence the fulfillment of the central purpose.[7]

The Central Purpose

"The nurse's central purpose defines the quality of health she desires to effect or sustain in her patient and specifies what she recognizes to be her special responsibility in caring for him."[8] This central purpose (or commitment) is based on the individual nurse's philosophy.

The nurse must believe in certain values and must express them by her actions and attitudes when working with patients. Wiedenbach identifies three essential components for a nursing philosophy: (1) a reverence for the gift of life; (2) a respect for the dignity, worth,

---

*Wiedenbach consistently uses the term *patient* and refers to the nurse as *her* in all her writings. This approach will be used in this chapter.

autonomy, and individuality of each human being; and (3) a resolution to act dynamically in relation to one's beliefs.[9] Any of these concepts might be further developed. However, Wiedenbach emphasizes the second in her work.

Wiedenbach's second concept is emphasized as she discusses the needed respect for the individual. She believes:

1. Each human being is endowed with unique potential to develop within himself the resources that enable him to maintain and sustain himself.
2. The human being basically strives toward self-direction and relative independence, and desires not only to make the best use of his capabilities and potentialities but to fulfill his responsibilities as well.
3. The human being needs stimulation in order to make the best use of his capabilities and realize his self-worth.
4. Whatever the individual does represents his best judgment at the moment of doing it.[10]

The Prescription

Once the nurse has identified her own philosophy and recognizes that the patient has autonomy and individuality, she can work *with* the individual to develop a *prescription* or plan for his care.

A *prescription* is a directive to activity.[11] A prescription may indicate the broad general action appropriate to implementation of the basic concepts, as well as suggest the kind of behavior needed to carry out these actions in accordance with the central purpose. These actions may be voluntary or involuntary. Voluntary action is an intended response, whereas involuntary action is an unintended response.[12]

A prescription is a directive to at least three kinds of voluntary action: (1) *mutually understood and agreed upon* action (the practitioner has evidence that the recipient understands the implications of the intended action and is psychologically and/or physiologically receptive to it); (2) *recipient-directed* action (the recipient of the action essentially directs the way it is to be carried out); and (3) *practitioner-directed* action (the practitioner carries out the action).[13] The prescription, according to Wiedenbach, specifies both the nature of the action that will most likely lead to fulfillment of the nurse's central purpose in nursing and the thinking process that determines it.

The Realities

When the nurse has determined her central purpose and has developed the prescription, then she must consider the *realities* of the situation in which she is to provide nursing care.

Wiedenbach defines the *realities* of the immediate situation as "the matrix within which the action occurs."[14] There are five realities as identified below:

1. The *agent*, practicing nurse or her delegate, characterized by her personal attributes, her capacities, her capabilities, and most importantly, her commitment and competence in nursing.
2. The *recipient*, who is the patient, characterized by his personal attributes, his problems, his capacities, his aspirations, and most importantly, his ability to cope with the concerns or problems he is experiencing.
3. The *goal*, which is the end to be attained through nursing action.
4. The *means*, which constitute the method, involving application of knowledge and of spiritual and material resources essential for the attainment of the goal.
5. The *framework*, consisting of the human, environmental, professional, and organizational facilities that not only make up the context within which nursing is practiced but also constitute its currently existing limits.[15]

The realities offer uniqueness to every situation. The success of professional nursing practice is dependent on them. Unless the realities are recognized and are dealt with, they may prevent the achievement of the goal.

Central purpose, prescription, and realities (components of prescriptive theory) are interdependent on one another as depicted in Figure 10-1. The prescription is derived by the nurse from her central purpose and is affected by the realities of the situation. The nurse develops a prescription based on her central purpose, which is implemented in the realities of the situation. Together these components constitute the substance of Wiedenbach's prescriptive theory. This theory when articulated serves as the guiding light of professional practice.[16]

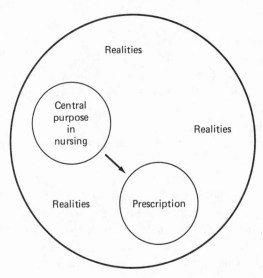

Figure 10-1. Wiedenbach's prescriptive theory. [*Adapted from* Ernestine Wiedenbach, *Meeting the Realities in Clinical Teaching* New York: Springer Publishing Company, Inc., 1969), p. x.]

WIEDENBACH'S CONCEPTUALIZATION OF THE NURSING PROCESS

The quality of nursing is measured by the nurse's actions, which elicit the behavioral and physiological responses from the patient that are in accordance with the nurse's central purpose. A nursing action is the visible portion of nursing practice in which the nurse interacts by word, look, manner, or deed with another person—e.g., the patient or another member of the patient's family—to bring about the desired result. A nursing action may be viewed as an "energized phenomenon"—one that occurs within the realities of the existing situation. There is a series of operations underlying and powering each action, operations that give each action impact and direction. This series constitutes the nursing process.[17]

The nursing process is essentially an internal personalized mechanism. As such, it is influenced by the nurse's culture, purpose in nursing, knowledge, wisdom, and sensitivity.[18]

In Wiedenbach's nursing process (see Figure 10-2) she identifies seven levels of awareness: sensation, perception, assumption, realization, insight, design, and decision.[19] The nursing process begins with an activating situation. This situation exists among the realities and serves as a stimulus to arouse the nurse's consciousness. This consciousness leads to a subjective interpretation of the first three levels, which are defined as: *sensation* (experienced sensory impression), *perception* (the interpretation of a sensory impression), and *assumption* (the meaning the nurse attaches to the perception). These three levels of awareness are obtained through the focus of the nurse's attention on the stimulus; they are intuitive rather than cognitive, and may initiate an involuntary response.

For example, a nurse enters a patient's room and states, "My, it's hot in here!" She immediately goes to the window and opens it. The *sensation* is: the room temperature. The *perception* is: "It feels hot." The *assumption* is: "If I am hot, then the patient must be hot." The involuntary response is to open the window.

Progressing from intuition to cognition, the nurse's actions become voluntary rather than involuntary. The next four levels of awareness occur in the voluntary phase. These are: *realization* (in which the nurse begins to validate the assumption she had previously made about the patient's behavior); *insight* (which includes joint planning and additional knowledge about the cause of the problem); *design* (the plan of action decided upon by the nurse and confirmed by the patient); and *decision* (the nurse's performance of a responsible action).[20]

To continue with the previous example: The nurse asks, "Are you too warm?" and the patient replies, "No, I'm not. I have felt cold since I washed my hair." The nurse responds, "I will close the window and get you a blanket." The patient agrees, "That would be fine." The nurse shuts the window and gets a blanket for the patient.

The *realization* is: the validation of the patient's perception of warmth. The *insight* is: the additional information that the patient had washed his hair. The *design* is: the plan to close the window and get a blanket as confirmed by the patient. The *decision* is: the nurse shuts the window and gets a blanket for the patient.

COMPARISON OF WIEDENBACH'S THEORY AND THE NURSING PROCESS

Comparing Wiedenbach's theory to the nursing process as defined in Chapter 2 indicates there is some degree of similarity, and many significant differences.

Assessment considers the patient holistically and requires extensive data collection. In Wiedenbach's model (see Figure 10-2) the nurse is stimulated, then assesses at the sensation and perception levels, levels that are involuntary and intuitive. The nurse makes an assumption about the situation and may act involuntarily. Such acts

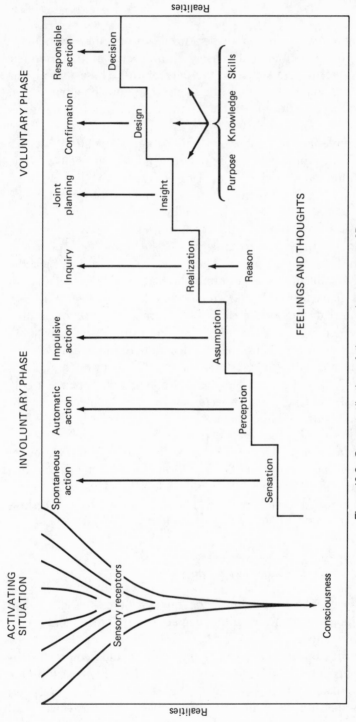

Figure 10-2. Conceptualization of the nursing process. [*Reproduced from* Joy P. Clausen and others. *Maternity Nursing Today* (New York: McGraw-Hill Book Company, 1977), p. 43.]

are spontaneous, automatic, or impulsive. They occur on the spur of the moment and are precipitated by unchecked, rampant thoughts and feelings. Occasionally in an emergency they may be lifesaving. However, these involuntary acts are more likely to do harm than good.[21]

In the nursing process, the *nursing diagnosis* is made after much conscious thought and deliberation about the assessment data. In Wiedenbach's model the assumption that can be compared to the nursing diagnosis is made on an intuitive level. This assumption should be validated by gathering more data. This validation occurs in Wiedenbach's realization level, which is voluntary and involves conscious thought. Once the assumption has been validated, the nurse may continue to gather more assessment data about the cause of the problem on the insight level. This may be considered *reassessment* as defined in Chapter 2.

Planning, the third phase of the nursing process, can be compared to Wiedenbach's levels of insight and design, which are part of her voluntary phase. The insight level of this model includes joint planning. This level is defined as joint planning between the nurse and the patient and does not involve other health care professionals.

Wiedenbach does not directly incorporate the concept of goal as part of the nursing process. However, she identifies goal in the context of her prescriptive theory as a component of the nurse's central purpose.[22] In the design level the nurse plans a course of action. After the plan is decided on, the nurse confirms it with the patient. Once the plan has been decided on and confirmed, the nurse performs the action. This level is comparable to the *implementation* phase.

In Wiedenbach's model of the nursing process she does not identify the *evaluation* phase. She alludes to evaluation when she states that nursing practice is directed toward "validation that the help provided was indeed helpful to the patient."[23]

WIEDENBACH AND THE CONCEPTS OF MAN, HEALTH, SOCIETY, AND NURSING

Wiedenbach emphasizes that the human being possesses unique potential, strives toward self-direction, needs stimulation, and whatever the individual does represents his best judgment at that moment. She believes these characteristics require respect from the nurse.[24]

The nurse's central purpose determines that her role will be that of a helper.[25] Nursing is the application of knowledge and skill toward meeting a need for help expressed by a patient. Nursing is a helping process with action directed toward providing something the patient requires or desires, a process that will restore or extend the patient's ability to cope with demands implicit in his healthy situation.[26]

Wiedenbach does not define the concept of health. However, she supports the World Health Organization's definition of health as a state of complete physical, mental, and social well-being and not merely the absence of disease and infirmity.[27]

Also, Wiedenbach does not discuss the concept of society. In her work she refers to the nurse as giving care to an individual and meeting that individual's needs.

SUMMARY

Wiedenbach identifies three concepts in her nursing theory, which she terms a *prescriptive theory*. These concepts of *central purpose, prescription,* and *realities* are interrelated to form her theory. The central purpose is the nurse's philosophy for care; the prescription is the directive to activity; the realities are the matrix in which the action occurs. The interrelationship of these concepts into her theory would be as follows: The nurse develops a prescription based on her central purpose, which is implemented in the realities of the situation.

Wiedenbach's conceptualization of the nursing process has three phases: (1) activating situation, (2) involuntary phase, and (3) voluntary phase.[28] The stimulus causes an involuntary response, which progresses to a voluntary response or the nurse's action. The levels within the involuntary phase are sensation, perception, and assumption. The levels within the voluntary phase are realization, insight, design, and decision. The entire nursing process occurs within the realities.

There are marked differences when Wiedenbach's nursing process is compared with the five-phase nursing process discussed in Chapter 2. Wiedenbach's *assessment* is reflexive and intuitive. The *nursing diagnosis* is made by assumption and is then validated. The patient is involved in the *planning* of his care. The nurse decides the care to be given, the patient confirms the plan, and the nurse does the *implementation*. Wiedenbach does not directly identify the phase of *evaluation*.

When comparing Wiedenbach's theory with the basic characteristics of theories outlined in Chapter 1, it meets the following criteria: interrelation of concepts in such a way as to create a different way of looking at a particular phenomenon; logical in nature; and contributes to and assists in increasing the general body of knowledge within the discipline. However, it would be difficult to validate or to test the theory by research.

Ernestine Wiedenbach was practicing nursing in the 1920s. She was a pioneer in the writing of nursing theory. Her work contributes significantly to the development of nursing as a profession.

NOTES

1. Ernestine Wiedenbach, *Clinical Nursing, A Helping Art* (New York: Springer Publishing Company, Inc., 1964), p. 1.
2. Joy P. Clausen and others, *Maternity Nursing Today* (New York: McGraw-Hill Book Company, 1977), p. 39.
3. Ibid.
4. Wiedenbach, *Clinical Nursing*, p. 2.
5. James Dickoff, Patricia A. James, and Ernestine Wiedenbach, "Theory in a Practice Discipline II: Practice-Orientated Research," *Nursing Research*, 17 (November-December 1968), 545-554.
6. Ernestine Wiedenbach, *Meeting the Realities in Clinical Teaching* (New York: Springer Publishing Company, Inc., 1969).
7. Ibid., p. 2.
8. Wiedenbach, *Clinical Nursing*, p. 16.
9. Ibid.
10. Ibid., p. 17.
11. Wiedenbach, *Meeting the Realities*, p. 3.
12. Ibid., p. 3.
13. Ibid.
14. Ibid., p. 4.
15. Clausen and others, *Maternity Nursing Today*, pp. 5-6.
16. Wiedenbach, *Meeting the Realities*, p. 5.
17. Clausen and others, *Maternity Nursing Today*, p. 41.
18. Ibid., p. 44.
19. Ibid., pp. 41-44.
20. Ibid.
21. Ibid., p. 42.
22. Wiedenbach, *Meeting the Realities*, p. 95.
23. Clausen and others, *Maternity Nursing Today*, p. 39.

24. Wiedenbach, *Clinical Nursing*, p. 17.
25. Ibid., p. 36.
26. Ibid.
27. Clausen and others, *Maternity Nursing Today*, p. 39.
28. Ibid., p. 43.

REFERENCES

Books

CLAUSEN, JOY, and others, *Maternity Nursing Today*. New York: McGraw-Hill Book Company, 1977.

NURSING DEVELOPMENT CONFERENCE GROUP, *Concept Formalization in Nursing*. Boston: Little, Brown & Company, 1973.

WIEDENBACH, ERNESTINE, *Clinical Nursing, A Helping Art*. New York: Springer Publishing Company, Inc., 1964.

———, *Family-Centered Maternity Nursing*. New York: G. P. Putnam's Sons, 1967.

———, *Meeting the Realities in Clinical Teaching*. New York: Springer Publishing Company, Inc., 1969.

Articles

DICKOFF, JAMES J., "Symposium in Theory Development in Nursing, Researching Research's Role in Theory Development," *Nursing Research*, 17 (May-June 1968), 204–206.

DICKOFF, JAMES J. and PATRICIA A. JAMES, "Symposium of Theory Development in Nursing: A Theory of Theories: A Position Paper," *Nursing Research*, 17 (May-June 1968), 197–203.

DICKOFF, JAMES J., and E. WIEDENBACH, "Theory in a Practice Discipline I: Practice-Orientated Discipline," *Nursing Research*, 17 (September-October 1968), 415–435.

DICKOFF, JAMES J., PATRICIA A. JAMES, and ERNESTINE WIEDENBACH, "Theory in a Practice Discipline II: Practice-Orientated Research," *Nursing Research*, 17 (November-December 1968), 545–554.

WIEDENBACH, E., "Childbirth as Mothers Say They Like It," *Public Health Nursing*, 51 (August 1949), 417–421.

———, "Nurse-Midwifery, Purpose, Practice and Opportunity," *Nursing Outlook*, 8 (May 1960), 256.

———, "The Helping Art of Nursing," *American Journal of Nursing*, 63 (November 1963), 54–57.

————, "Family Nurse Practitioner for Maternal and Child Care," *Nursing Outlook*, 13 (December 1965), 50 ff.

————, "Genetics and the Nurse," *Bulletin of the American College of Nurse Midwifery*, 13 (May 1968), 8–13.

————, "The Nurse's Role in Family Planning—A Conceptual Base for Practice," *Nursing Clinics of North America*, 3 (June 1968), 355 ff.

————, "Nurses' Wisdom in Nursing Theory," *American Journal of Nursing*, 70 (May 1970), 1057 ff.

————, "Comment on Beliefs and Values: Basis for Curriculum Design," *Nursing Research*, 19 (September-October 1970), 427.

11

MYRA ESTRIN LEVINE

Connie Hetrick Esposito and Mary Kathryn Leonard

Myra E. Levine received her nursing education in three institutions: Cook County School of Nursing, Chicago; B.S., University of Chicago; and M.S.N., Wayne State University, Detroit, Michigan. Her nursing experience includes staff nursing, administrative and teaching supervision, clinical instruction, and direction of nursing services. She was chairman of the Department of Clinical Nursing at Cook County School of Nursing. She has also held positions as Associate Professor of Nursing, College of Nursing, University of Illinois, Chicago; faculty member at Loyola University School of Nursing, Chicago; and Director of Continuing Education, Evanston Hospital, Evanston, Illinois.

Mrs. Levine is the author of a number of articles that have been published in nursing journals and of one book dealing with nursing (see references at end of chapter). In 1965 she presented a paper at the Regional Clinical Conferences sponsored by the American Nurses' Association. This paper, "Trophicogenosis: An Alternative to Nursing Diagnosis," can be found in the American Nurses' Association publication Exploring Progress in Medical-Surgical Nursing Practice, *New York, 1966, Vol. 2. In addition, Mrs. Levine has participated in a number of workshops and conferences.*

She is a member of Sigma Theta Tau (Alpha Beta Chapter,

Loyola University), a Charter Fellow of the American Academy of Nursing, and an honorary member of the American Mental Health Aid to Israel. She is listed in Who's Who of American Women *and received the Elizabeth Russell Belford Award for Education from Sigma Theta Tau in 1977.*

The development of Levine's theory of nursing reflects an integration of the various theories and concepts presented in the sciences and humanities that have influenced trends in nursing. There are four scientific concepts/theories that have had the greatest impact on the development of nursing trends. These are: the great healing concept, the germ theory, the theory of multiple factors, and the unified theory of health and disease.

According to the great healing concept, nature would take its course and healing would occur. Influenced by this concept, Nightingale theorized that nursing should focus on providing the individual with a supportive environment to enhance nature's work of healing.[1]

Nightingale never fully accepted the germ theory. This theory identified a direct relationship between germs and disease and/or illness. Nursing at this time followed the lead of medicine and began to focus on disease causation and treatment. The thrust of nursing education was skill training for the implementation of procedures and treatments.

The theory of multiple factors introduced the idea that illness was a result of a combination of factors rather than just a germ.[2] The multiple factors theory was supported by Maslow's hierarchy of needs, which theorized that the healthy individual must sufficiently satisfy increasingly more complex physiological and psychological needs.[3]

Gradually nursing shifted its focus from skill training and procedures to total patient care, i.e., to meeting the psychological as well as the physical needs of the patient. The concept of total patient care was introduced by Lydia Hall.[4]

The unified theory of health and disease has been influenced by the concept of holism and the proposition of a health-illness continuum.[5] This continuum suggests the existence of a sliding scale of individual health conditions ranging from health to illness. The systems theory premise, that the whole is greater than the sum of its parts, further supports the holism concept. Thus, the trend toward total patient care still remains today.

Within this framework of total patient care, Levine has developed four conservation principles that serve as the basis of her nursing theory (see p. 153). This theory focuses the nurse's implementation on the patient's adaptation and response to illness.

This chapter will include a discussion of Levine's theory of nursing, its application to the nursing process, and the relationship of the concepts of humanity, society, health, nursing, and learning. A brief case study is included to demonstrate the application of this theory.

LEVINE'S THEORY OF NURSING

In order to understand Levine's theory of nursing, it is necessary to consider her definition of nursing. Levine's definition of nursing makes three assumptions: (1) Nursing is human interaction.[6] (2) Nursing is a discipline based on the idea that people are dependent on their relationships with other people.[7] (3) Nursing is based on intervention that supports or promotes the patient's adjustment.[8]

There are four major components to Levine's theory.

1. The patient is in the predicament of illness.
2. The nurse must recognize the organismic manifestation of the patient's adaptation to illness.
3. The patient's environment includes the nurse.
4. The nurse, who must recognize the organismic response of the patient, must make an intervention in the patient's environment and must evaluate the intervention as therapeutic or supportive.[9]

Levine's theory next makes three basic assumptions about the nurse-patient interaction. These assumptions on which interactions are based are determined by (1) the *conditions* in which the patient enters the health care setting, (2) the *functions* of the nurse in the situation, and (3) the *responsibilities* of the nurse in the situation. The patient entering the health care setting is in a state of altered health or illness. The nurse interacting with the patient has the responsibility of recognizing the patient's organismic response, intervening to promote the patient's adaptation to the state of illness, and evaluating the intervention as being supportive or therapeutic. *Organismic response* is changes in behavior or changes in level of functioning of the body exhibited by the person adapting or attempting to adapt to the environment.

Adaptation is the process of adjusting or modifying behavior or functioning to fit the situation.

The nurse is expected to base both therapeutic and supportive interventions on scientific or theoretical knowledge. This theory assumes that the nurse is able to make the necessary judgments to promote or support the patient's adaptation based on knowledge. In addition, the nurse is expected to possess the skill necessary to implement these interventions.

Nursing interventions may be to support the patient to adapt to a level of altered health. In the case of a patient with terminal illness, intervention will not help to restore the patient to a state of health, but certain interventions will help to maintain the patient's present state of altered health and to prevent further health deterioration. These nursing interventions are referred to as *supportive interventions*. For the patient who is not terminally ill, the nurse has the responsibility to promote the patient's adaptation in a way that leads to the patient's return to a state of health. Nursing interventions that promote healing and restoration of health are referred to as *therapeutic interventions*.

Conservation Principles

The person is viewed holistically by Levine as requiring structural, personal, and social integrity as well as energy to be in a state of health. If any of these elements is disrupted or changed, the person is in a state of altered health (illness). All nursing interventions are based on the conservation of these four elements. The term *conservation* in Levine's theory means to keep together or maintain a proper balance.[10] Levine labels nursing activities as *nursing interventions*. Patient activities involve the patient's participation in his/her care within the safe limits of his/her ability to do so.[11] The purpose of the conservation is to maintain the unity and integrity of the patient. The four principles are as follows: (1) *Conservation of energy* refers to balancing energy output and energy input to avoid excessive fatigue, i.e., adequate rest, nutrition, and exercise. (2) *Conservation of structural integrity* refers to maintaining or restoring the structure of the body, i.e., prevention of physical breakdown and the promotion of healing. (3) *Conservation of personal integrity* refers to maintenance or restoration of the patient's sense of identity and self-worth, i.e., acknowledgement of uniqueness. (4) *Conservation of social integrity* refers to the acknowledgement of the patient as a social being. It involves the recognition and presentation of human interaction, particularly with the patient's significant others.[12]

Example. The following is an example of how Levine's theory could be utilized. Tommy is ten years old. He is hospitalized with a disorder of the gastro-intestinal tract. He exhibits nausea, vomiting, and diarrhea as well as a decreased activity level. Based on these signs (organismic response), the nurse recognizes Tommy's body is attempting to adjust to illness. Using the principles of conservation as the theoretical base, the nurse makes interventions in Tommy's environment (see Table 11-1).

The nurse observes Tommy to see how he is adjusting to his altered state of health *with* the nursing interventions. Tommy's nausea, vomiting, and diarrhea decrease. The skin around his anal area remains intact. He is up more and actively participates in the selection of clear liquids. He plays checkers with his father and laughs when he wins. Based on these observations the nurse decides what, if any, further nursing interventions are needed.

LEVINE'S THEORY
AND THE NURSING PROCESS

Levine's theory for nursing parallels many elements of the nursing process. According to Levine the nurse must observe the patient, decide on an appropriate intervention, perform it, and then evaluate its usefulness in helping the patient. Also, Levine's theory assumes the nurse and patient will participate together in the patient's care. However, the nursing process described in Chapter 2 emphasizes more mutuality between the patient and the nurse than is implied in Levine's theory. In Levine's theory the patient is assumed to be in a dependent position. As a result of this dependent position the patient is in need of nursing assistance to help in adaptation toward a state of health. The nursing process, on the other hand, does not necessarily assume the client is in a dependent position. At this point, the steps of the nursing process and their relationship to Levine's theory will be discussed specifically.

In the *assessment* phase, the patient is assessed using basically two methods: interviewing and observation. The focus is on the patient; the family and/or significant others are only considered from the perspective of how they might help or interfere with the patient's well-being. The needs of the family and/or significant others are not considered in relation to the patient. According to Levine, if a family member's needs are going to be dealt with, that person must become the target of the assessment.

In performing the holistic assessment, the nurse uses Levine's four conservation principles as an assessment guide. The nurse is concerned with the patient's balance of energy and maintenance of integrity. Thus, the nurse collects data about the patient's energy sources, i.e., nutrition, sleep-rest, leisure, coping patterns, significant

Table 11-1

Application of Levine's Theory
to a Given Example

Intervention	Conservation Principle	Therapeutic/ Supportive	Rationale
1. Tommy is allowed up as tolerated.	1. Energy	1. Therapeutic	1. Attempt to restore energy balance.
2. Tommy is allowed to drink two ounces of clear liquid each hour.	2. (A) Energy (B) Structural integrity	2. (A) Therapeutic (B) Supportive	2. (A) Attempt to restore energy balance. (B) Prevent skin breakdown from inadequate hydration.
3. Instruct Tommy to wash and dry his anal area after each stool.	3. Structural integrity	3. Supportive	3. Prevent breakdown of skin in anal area.
4. Tommy is encouraged to select the flavor of the clear liquid each hour.	4. Personal integrity	4. Supportive	4. Maintain individuality and autonomy.
5. Tommy's sister and parents are encouraged to play board games with him during visitation.	5. (A) Social integrity (B) Energy	5. (A) Supportive (B) Therapeutic	5. (A) Maintain Tommy's relationship with family members. (B) Attempt to restore energy balance.

relationships, medications, and environment. Data are also collected about the expenditures of energy, i.e., the functioning of various body systems, emotional and/or social stresses, and work patterns. In addition, data are collected about the patient's structural integrity, i.e., body defenses and physical body structure. In the area of personal integrity, data are collected about the patient's self-system, i.e., uniqueness, values, religious beliefs, and economic resources. Lastly, in the area of social integrity, data are collected about the decision-making processes of the patient, the patient's relationships with others, and his involvement in social/community affairs.

After the collection of all the data, the nurse critically analyzes the data to obtain a holistic view of the patient. This analysis reflects the patient's balance of strengths and weaknesses in each of the four assessment areas (conservation principles). The analysis also identifies areas needing further data collection. In the analysis, concepts and theories from other disciplines are also considered. Levine's theory has a close kinship to Maslow's hierarchy of needs and Selye's stress theory.[13] In Selye's stress theory there is a stressor that stimulates a response as part of the general adaptation syndrome. In Levine's theory illness is the stressor and the patient is continually trying to adapt to this changed state. This adaptation is manifested in the patient's organismic response, which includes changes in behavior or levels of functioning of the body.

Levine's theory also supports the work and beliefs of Florence Nightingale in relation to her concept of environment (see Chapter 3). Nursing has the responsibility of providing a supportive environment, one that is conducive to health and healing. In Levine's theory the nurse is part of the patient's environment.

From the analysis the nurse develops a *nursing diagnosis*. Since the patient is in a state of illness or altered health, the nursing diagnosis will reflect a problem or potential problem related to a deficit or a threatened deficit in one of the four areas of conservation. Levine's theory does not make provision for health promotion needs/teaching. The provision for health promotion is limited to areas directly related to the patient's present problem(s) associated with the illness and/or state of altered health. Therefore, it may be concluded that the nurse utilizing this theory has a time orientation in the present. Thus the nurse is not concerned with future planning except as it relates to the patient's present problem.

In the *planning* phase, which includes goal setting, the nursing process emphasizes the mutuality of this activity between nurse and patient. Levine, however, has not specifically indicated or stressed the need for mutual goal setting. It may be concluded that mutuality was not intended in her theory. The data that support this assumption are: (1) the dependent position of the patient as a result of the state of illness and/or altered health with need for nursing assistance, and (2) the nurse's responsibility to monitor the patient's condition in order to regulate the balance between nursing intervention and patient participation in care. The nurse, as an individual, may include the patient in this activity based on the nurse's assessment of the patient's ability to participate in the goal-setting activity. In order for these goals to be workable, the nurse states the goal in behavioral terms so it is measurable. The goals reflect an attempt to help the patient adapt and reach a state of health.

Also, in the *planning* phase, the nurse uses the goal (1) to determine the strategies to be used in the plan and (2) to determine the extent to which the plan must be developed to meet the goal. Levine indicated the nurse bases practice on knowledge. Thus, the steps of the nursing plan would be based on principles, laws, concepts, and theories from the sciences and humanities. Also in developing the plan, the nurse considers the patient's ability to participate in the plan of care, and the patient's degree of participation is identified. During the planning phase, the nurse may consult with other health care team members.

As the plan of care is *implemented*, the nurse observes the patient for an organismic response. Data are collected and are used later in the evaluation phase. During the implementation phase, the nurse is responsible for the care given to the patient. Levine's theory indicates that (1) the nurse is expected to possess the skill necessary to carry out the nursing interventions, and (2) the nursing interventions are aimed at supporting or promoting the patient's adaptation.

In the *evaluation* phase, the nurse considers the organismic response of the patient to the nursing action. The nurse uses the data collected about the patient's organismic response to determine if the nursing intervention was therapeutic or supportive. If the intervention was therapeutic, the patient is adapting and is progressing toward a state of health. Levine did not indicate that an overall evaluation of the patient's progress was needed. However, in using the nursing process the nurse would make an evaluative determination about the patient's progress toward or away from goal achievement. The data collected in the evaluation would be included in the assessment, and the nursing process would be repeated if needed.

Levine's theory lends itself to use in the nursing process. However, one must remember that in using Levine's theory the focus of the process is on one person, the time orientation is the present, and the patient is in a dependent position and in an altered or impaired state of health.

RELATIONSHIP TO OTHER CONCEPTS

Levine's theory of nursing can be related to five major concepts: humanity, society, health, learning, and nursing. Levine views the *individual* as dependent on his relationship with others. This becomes particularly apparent in the principle of conservation of social integrity. The relationships of the patient with his/her significant others are important enough for Levine to focus on restoring or maintaining the balance between them. *Humanity* is viewed as an individual patient trying to adjust to an altered state of health. The principle of conservation of personal integrity lends itself to the idea of attempting to adjust in response to a state of illness. The self-worth of the patient is the focus. The individual is also viewed as exhibiting behavior changes and/or changes in the level of functioning as attempts are made to adjust to the stress of illness (organismic response). The balance normally present in the holistic individual is disrupted by illness and shows in these changes. All the principles of conservation are aimed at restoring or maintaining the holistic balance of the individual.

Society is viewed broadly by Levine. Society is composed of the environment the patient experiences at any time. Levine makes a point of including the nurse in the patient's environment. In her theory the environment is the health care system. Society is also made up of the family and significant others. In discussing the conservation of social integrity, Levine briefly mentions all of society and the entire social system.[14]

Levine's theory relates to the concept of *health* in the sense of altered or disrupted health. Her theory only applies to people in a state of illness. Health practices are primarily considered as they relate to illness. Nursing care is directed toward the restoration of health. Only in discussing the whole social system does Levine make reference to preventive health practices as being desirable and worth pursuing.[15] However, since no further explanation is given, it is assumed that health must be altered for one to participate in her system.

Levine's theory relates to the concept of *learning* in a variety of ways. In order to make nursing interventions based on theory and knowledge, one has to first learn them. In the example of Tommy, there are many theories and scientific knowledges required. A knowledge of communication and interaction theory is basic. The nurse must also know the anatomy and physiology of the gastrointestinal tract—structure, motility, and gastric secretions and their actions. A knowledge of nutrition, fluid and electrolyte balance, and anatomy and physiology of the skin is necessary. Growth and developmental theories are appropriate for selection of specific activities that fit Tommy and his developmental tasks. Tommy's responses to the stresses of illness and hospitalization can be observed by assessing his general adaptation system. In addition, separation from family and home is usually stressful. This makes it important for the nurse to utilize stress and adaptation theories to help Tommy deal with his present situation. Need theory is used to identify and meet Tommy's needs. Evaluation theory is used to make a judgment about the nursing interventions. The reader can probably select even more theories that relate to Tommy and his care.

It is important to note that Maslow's hierarchy of needs has been utilized by Levine in the development of her theory. The conservation principles incorporate all but one of the hierarchy of needs. Energy conservation deals with physiologic and safety needs. Conservation of structural integrity deals with physiologic needs also. The belonging and love needs are dealt with through the conservation of personal integrity, and needs for self-esteem are dealt with in the conservation of social integrity.[16] There is much learning involved in the understanding and utilization of Levine's theory.

Levine's theory relates to the concept of *nursing* because it is an approach to the giving of nursing care. It involves some basic assumptions, as follows: (1) human interaction is paramount for nursing to take place. (2) The nurse must possess both skills and a theoretical and scientific knowledge base. (3) Nursing is based on the assessment or recognition of behavioral changes and/or changes in the level of functioning of the patient during efforts to adapt in response to illness.

THEORY VERSUS CONCEPT

The first criterion for a theory is that it can interrelate concepts in such a manner as to create a different way of looking at a particular phenomenon. In considering Levine's ideas about nursing, the concepts of illness, adaptation, nursing interventions, and evaluation of nursing interventions are interrelated in just that way. They are combined to look at nursing care in a different way (perhaps a more comprehensive view incorporating total patient care) from previous times.

A theory must be logical in nature. Levine's ideas about nursing are organized in such a way as to be sequential and logical. They can be used to explain the consequences of nursing actions. There are no apparent contradictions in her ideas.

A theory can be used as the basis for development of hypotheses that can be tested. Levine's ideas can be tested. Hypotheses can be derived from them. The ideas lend themselves to being tested. The principles of conservation are specific enough to be testable with the exception of the conservation of social integrity. For example, it is possible to test if physiologic structure is being supported or improved, thus testing the principle of conservation of structural integrity.

The fourth criterion is that a theory contributes to and assists in increasing the general body of knowledge within the discipline through the research implemented to validate it. Since Levine's ideas have not yet been widely researched, it is hard to determine a contribution to the general body of knowledge within the discipline.

Chapter 1 indicates the most significant characteristic of a theory is its usefulness to the practitioner. Levine's ideas can be used by practitioners to guide and improve their practice. These ideas lend themselves to use in practice, particularly the acute care setting.

The last criterion for a theory is that it must be consistent with other validated theories, laws, and principles. Levine's ideas seem to be consistent with other theories, laws and principles. They support humanitarian knowledge and scientific principles. Since Levine's ideas meet four of the six criteria for a theory, one can designate them as a theory of nursing. Levine herself does not refer to her ideas as either theory or concept.

CONCLUSIONS

Levine's theory for nursing focuses on one person—the patient. In utilizing this theory the nurse is concerned with the patient's family and/or significant others only to the point that they influence or have an effect on the patient's progress. Thus, the utilization of this theory is limited. This theory could not be used in working with families, groups, or communities.

Levine's theory recognizes nursing as a profession whose practice is based on scientific knowledge and skill. Her theory implies that nursing is considered as an independent practice profession. No mention is made about the relationship of nursing to the other health care professions. This theory does not make provisions for preventive teaching or anticipatory guidance, which are considered to be nursing functions. These limitations may influence the collaboration with other health care team members. Continuity of care and long-range planning for the patient are limited by the omission of anticipatory guidance and preventive teaching in the area of health promotion. As mentioned before, provisions are made for anticipatory guidance and health teaching only as they relate to the patient's present illness.

Levine's theory for nursing is compatible with the practice of nursing in an acute care setting. The theory emphasizes the dependent position of the patient, the patient's impaired state of health, the patient's limited participation in his/her own care, and the increased responsibility of the nurse in directing and coordinating the patient's care. Thus, one might assume that these conditions are most likely to exist in a critical care unit or in an emergency care area. Levine's theory has definite limitations for utilization in other areas where the focus is on long-term care and rehabilitation. The time orientation is to the present. A present-time orientation limits the attention that can be focused on health promotion and illness prevention. The practice of preventive health care and more specifically health promotion assume an interest in or a concern for anticipating future needs. Thus, in a program or course that is health-oriented, Levine's theory would be philosophically incompatible.

Levine's theory speaks to the patient's sense of personal integrity, i.e., autonomy and uniqueness. In the illness state, the patient is placed in a dependent position. This placement of the patient may clearly threaten the individual's sense of autonomy. This is a particular area of concern. In this theory the nurse has the responsibility for determining the patient's ability to participate in the care given and for maintaining the balance between this participation and nursing intervention. If the perceptions of the nurse and the patient about the patient's ability to participate in care do not match, then this mismatch will be an area of conflict. From this placement of the client in a dependent position, one may conclude that the client is not viewed as a member of the health care team. Also, one may question if Levine's theory is not incongruent. If an individual has personal integrity, can the individual be given limited autonomy or be placed in a dependent position?

Finally, Levine's theory reflects the current beliefs about the holistic nature of humanity. However, within the theory there is some obscurity about definitions of the conservation principles, particularly social integrity. The utility of this theory for nursing in the future is questionable if the trend is toward the nurse's increased responsibility in health promotion and preventive health teaching.

SUMMARY

In Levine's theory of nursing, nursing is human interaction. This is based on the idea that people are dependent on their relationships with others. The nurse has the responsibility to intervene in the patient's situation after recognizing the patient's organismic response. Nursing interventions are supportive (maintain the status quo) or therapeutic (promote healing and restoration). The nurse's interventions are based on the four conservation principles. These are: (1) conservation of energy, (2) conservation of structural integrity, (3) conservation of personal integrity, and (4) conservation of social integrity. These conservation principles provide a guideline for viewing the individual in a holistic manner.

Levine's theory does relate to the concepts of humanity, society, health, learning, nursing, and the nursing process. Its major limitations relate to its focus on the individual, on illness, and on the dependency of the patient.

NOTES

1. Myra Estrin Levine, *Introduction to Clinical Nursing*, 2nd ed. (Philadelphia: F. A. Davis Co., 1973), pp. 4–5.
2. Ibid., p. 5.
3. A. H. Maslow, *Motivation and Personality* (New York: Harper and Row Publishers, Inc., 1954).
4. Lydia Hall, "Nursing—What is it?", *Virginia State Nurses' Association* (Winter 1959).
5. Levine, *Introduction to Clinical Nursing*, pp. 6–7.
6. Ibid., p. 1.
7. Ibid.
8. Ibid., p. 13.
9. Ibid., pp. 1–3.
10. Ibid., pp. 13–14.

11. Ibid., p. 13.
12. Ibid., pp. 14–18.
13. Maslow, *Motivation and Personality*; and Hans Selye, *The Stress of Life* (New York: McGraw-Hill Book Company, 1956), pp. 31–33.
14. Levine, *Introduction to Clinical Nursing*, p. 18.
15. Ibid.
16. Marjorie L. Byrne and Lida F. Thompson, *Key Concepts for the Study and Practice of Nursing* (St. Louis, Mo.: The C. V. Mosby Co., 1972), pp. 1–10; and Maslow, *Motivation and Personality*.

REFERENCES

BYRNE, MARJORIE L., and LIDA F. THOMPSON, *Key Concepts for the Study and Practice of Nursing*. St. Louis, Mo.: The C. V. Mosby Co., 1972.

LEVINE, MYRA E., "Adaptation and Assessment: A Rationale for Nursing Intervention," *American Journal of Nursing*, 66, no. 11 (November 1966), 2450–2453.

———, "Holistic Nursing," *Nursing Clinics of North America*, 6, no. 2 (June 1971), 253–264.

———, "The Intransigent Patient," *American Journal of Nursing*, 70, no. 10 (October 1970), 2106–2111.

———, *Introduction to Clinical Nursing*, 2nd ed. Philadelphia: F. A. Davis Co., 1973.

———, "The Four Conservation Principles of Nursing," *Nursing Forum*, VI, no. 1 (1967), 45–59.

NURSING DEVELOPMENT CONFERENCE GROUP, *Concept Formalization in Nursing: Process and Product*. Boston: Little, Brown & Company, 1973.

12

MARTHA E. ROGERS

Suzanne M. Falco and Marie L. Lobo

Martha E. Rogers was born in Dallas, Texas, May 12, 1914, the eldest of four children. Her family heritage includes many active women suffragists among her relatives and a strong belief in the necessity for a college education. Before entering the Knoxville General Hospital School of Nursing, she attended the University of Tennessee in Knoxville from 1931 to 1933. She received her diploma in 1936, a B.S. in public health nursing from George Peabody College, Nashville, Tennessee, in 1937; an M.A. in public health nursing supervision from Teachers College, Columbia University, New York, in 1945; and an M.P.H. in 1952 and a Sc.D. in 1954, both from Johns Hopkins University.

Following numerous leadership and staff positions in community health nursing, she moved into higher education as a visiting lecturer and then as a research associate. For twenty-one years, Dr. Rogers was Professor and Head of the Division of Nurse Education at New York University. Since 1975 she has continued to teach at the University.

Dr. Rogers has been active in numerous professional organizations, has received many awards and honors, and has published extensively in numerous nursing journals. She has authored several books.

As a humanistic science dedicated to compassionate concern for maintaining and promoting health, preventing illness, and caring for and rehabilitating the sick and disabled, nursing historically has meant service to humanity. Throughout nursing's evolution, from the earliest ages to the present, nurturance of the human race has been an ever-present and central concern.[1] Over the years, the scientific extension of people's centuries-long interest in life and its many manifestations have become integral components of nursing. Thus, the history of humanity is reflected in the evolutionary development of nursing. Consequently, Martha Rogers believes that knowledge of the past is a necessary foundation for the present understanding of nursing, and for evolving the theories and principles that must guide nursing practice.[2]

The concept that human life is valuable did not develop until people had begun to band together into tribes, villages, and towns. Such communal living allowed for sharing of work and responsibility and the provision of mutual support. This more settled life style made it possible for mothers to keep their newborns and care for more children.[3] Thus, partly out of love and partly out of need, human beings began to develop strong feelings about and concern for fellow human beings.

As culture developed and more complex concepts in economic, political, and social structures increased, the value of human life increased. Science, art, and religion brought a growing awareness of one's fellow human beings. The Hebrews developed a monotheistic faith, while the Greeks contributed philosophy, politics, and government. Humanism was becoming strongly entrenched in culture. Following the rise of Christianity, the medieval world was dominated by the Christian religions whose members assumed the responsibility for nursing. With the Dark Ages came a decline in religious, cultural, and political life. The end of this period led to the beginning of modern science.[4]

As modern science evolved, new ideas mushroomed into new discoveries. The nature of the universe was explored. Descartes established the basis of modern philosophy. Einstein's theory of relativity brought a fourth dimension in the coordinate of space-time to man's previously three-dimensional world. Space research has multiplied scientific knowledge and has altered life style. The reality of these evolutionary changes is reflected in man's growing complexity.

As a result of these factors, the rate at which society has been storing up useful knowledge about humanity and the universe has been spiraling upward for the past 10,000 years.[5] This vast storehouse of knowledge coupled with a high degree of humanism and value for life has made advancement of nursing through scientific means and theoretical development a reality.

ROGERS'S DEFINITION OF NURSING

Capitalizing on the knowledge base gained from anthropology, sociology, astronomy, religion, philosophy, history, and mythology, Rogers, in 1970, developed a conceptual framework for nursing. Since human beings are at the center of nursing's purpose, this conceptual framework for nursing looks at the total individual. Nursing, then, is a humanistic and a humanitarian science directed toward describing and explaining the human being in synergistic wholeness and in developing the hypothetical generalizations and predictive principles basic to knowledgeable practice. The science of nursing is a science of humanity—the study of the nature and direction of human development.[6]

BASIC ASSUMPTIONS

Underlying the conceptual framework developed by Rogers are five assumptions about human beings.[7] First, the human being is a unified whole possessing an individual integrity and manifesting characteristics that are more than and different from the sum of the parts. The distinctive properties of the whole are also significantly different from those of its parts. Extensive knowledge of the subsystems is ineffective in enabling one to determine the properties of the living system—the human being. The human being is visible only when particulars disappear from view. Because of this wholeness, the individual's life process is a dynamic course that is continuous, creative, evolutionary, and uncertain, resulting in highly variable and constantly changing patterning and organization.

Second, it is assumed that the individual and the environment are continuously exchanging matter and energy with each other. Environment for any individual is defined as the patterned wholeness of all that is external to a given individual. This constant interchange of materials and energy between the individual and the environment characterizes each of them as open systems.

The third assumption holds that the life process of human beings evolves irreversibly and unidirectionally along a space-time continuum. Consequently, the individual can never go backwards or be something he previously was. At any given point in time, then, the individual is the expression of the totality of events present at that given time.

Identifying individuals and reflecting their wholeness is life's pattern and organization. The pattern and organization allow for self-regulation, rhythmicity, and dynamism. They give unity to diversity and reflect a dynamic and creative universe. Thus, the fourth assumption is that pattern and organization identify individuals and reflect their innovative wholeness.

Finally, the fifth assumption is that the human being is characterized by the capacity for abstraction and imagery, language and thought, sensation and emotion. Of all the earth's life forms, only the human is a sentient, thinking being who perceives and ponders the vastness of the cosmos.

There is a strong parallel between Rogers's basic assumptions and general system theory. According to von Bertalanffy, a system is a set of elements standing in interrelations.[8] The interrelated elements in this conceptual model are human beings and their environments. As a living system, the individual is capable of taking in matter, energy, and information from the environment, and releasing matter, energy, and information to the environment.[9] Because of this exchange, the individual is an open system—an underlying assumption.

General system theory is a general science of wholeness. It is concerned with the problems of organization, phenomena that are not resolvable to individual events, and dynamic interactions manifested in the difference of the behavior of the parts when isolated. As a result, order and behavior are not understandable by investigation of the respective parts in isolation.[10] Thus, the assumption of wholeness results.

The principle of hierarchial order is applicable.[11] The individual as an open system attempts to move toward a higher order by progressive differentiation, as for example, the differentiation of the cells of the zygote to form a human being. Within the order of the universe, the human being is of a higher order than other two-legged animals. Characteristic of this is Rogers's fifth assumption of human beings as sentient, thinking beings.

Using these five assumptions as a base, the life process in human beings becomes a phenomenon of wholeness, of continuity, of dynamic and creative change. It possesses its own unity. It is inseparable from the environment. Since the individual is the recipient of nursing services, life processes of humanity are the *core* around which nursing revolves. According to Rogers, the science of nursing is directed toward describing the life process of humanity, and toward explaining and predicting the nature and direction of its development.[12]

ROGERS'S THEORY:
PRINCIPLES OF HOMEODYNAMICS

Although Rogers offers no theoretical statement, she grounded her *principles of homeodynamics* in the five basic assumptions as discussed above. The principles of homeodynamics are composed of three separate principles—complementarity, helicy, and resonancy.[13] Combining the principles of homeodynamics with the concept of humanity from her definition of nursing, a theoretical statement can be postulated. Using the definition that a theory states the relationship between concepts, an appropriate theoretical statement might be that nursing is the use of the principles of homeodynamics for the service of humanity.

Principles of Homeodynamics

The first principle is that of *complementarity*. Because of the inseparability of human beings and their environment, sequential changes in the life process are continuous revisions occurring from the interactions between human beings and their environment. Between the two entities, there is a constant mutual interaction and mutual change whereby simultaneous molding is taking place in both at the same time. Thus, complementarity is the continuous, mutual, simultaneous interaction process between human and environmental fields.

The next principle, *resonancy*, speaks to the nature of the change occurring between human and environmental fields. The change in the pattern and organization of human beings and environments is propagated by waves that move from lower frequency longer waves to higher frequency shorter waves. The life process in human beings is a symphony of rhythmical vibrations oscillating at various frequencies. Human beings experience their environments as a resonating wave of complex symmetry uniting them with the rest of the world. Resonancy, then, is the identification of the human field and the environmental field by wave patterns and organization manifesting continuous change from lower frequency longer waves to higher frequency shorter waves.

Finally, the principle of *helicy* states that the nature and direction of human and environmental changes are continuously innovative, probabilistic, and characterized by the increasing diversity of human field and environmental field pattern and organization emerging out of the continuous, mutual, simultaneous interaction between the human and environmental fields and manifesting nonrepeating rhythmicities. Because the life process is a constantly evolving series of changes in which the past has been incorporated and out of which new patterns have emerged, it is a becoming, a dynamic repatterning, a growing complexity, a unidirectional phenomenon, a probabilistic goal-directedness. The concepts of rhythmicality, evolutionary emergence, and the unitary nature of the human-environmental field relationship are encompassed. Therefore, helicy postulates the direction of the change occurring between the human and environmental fields.

Consequently, the principles of homeodynamics are a way of viewing human beings in their wholeness. Changes in the life process of humanity are irreversible, nonrepeatable, rhythmical in nature, and evidence of the growing complexity of pattern and organization. Change proceeds by continuous repatterning of both human and environmental fields by resonating oscillations of lower frequency longer waves to higher frequency shorter waves, and reflects the mutual simultaneous interaction between the two fields at any given point in space-time.

COMPARISON WITH OTHER THEORIES

The principles of homeodynamics are closely aligned to selected principles of general system theory. The homeodynamic principle of helicy can be compared to the principles of equifinality and negentropy. *Equifinality* means that an open system may attain a time-independent state independent of initial conditions and determined only by the system parameters. Thus, the system has a goal.[14] The *negentropic* principle provides that open systems have mechanisms that can slow down or arrest the process of movement toward less efficiency and growth.[15] Environmental exchange can provide support for such mechanisms.

For example, growth and development in the individual are equifinal. The same final state can be reached from different initial states and by means of different pathways. The various phases or stages along the way are maintained for an interval until spontaneous transition toward a higher order evokes new developments. The evolution toward an increase of order and organization at a higher level is made possible by negentropy.[16] Thus, growing complexity and evolutionary emergence are made possible.

Consider the case of identical twins Susie and Janie. Shortly after their two-month birthday, Susie spent six weeks in bilateral leg casts to correct a congenital deformity. As a result of this experience, Susie is maintained at a developmental plateau, while Janie continues to develop along the sequential axis. Consequently, Susie experiences a developmental lag. The extent of this lag is depicted in Figure 12-1. At four months, the lag is substantial, whereas at eight months the lag has been greatly reduced. The equifinal state of this development will be achieved, despite the increased time required.

Because of the evolutionary nature of this framework, many developmental theories are consistent with it. For example, Erikson's psychosocial stages of development beginning with trust vs. mistrust, and autonomy vs. shame and doubt, through generativity vs. self absorption and ego integrity vs. despair, profess a forward growth of an increasingly complex individual.[17] Havinghurst's developmental tasks support the same philosophy of growth and development as Erikson.[18] Development is an ongoing process from learning the first basic tasks of walking, eating, and talking to control of bodily functions to adjusting to retirement and/or death of a spouse. Another example is Piaget's concepts of intellectual development.[19] From sensorimotor to preoperational to concrete operational to formal operational thought, a nonreversible growth occurs. Kohlberg validates Piaget's work in his findings that moral development begins when thought processes shift from preoperational to concrete operations.[20] Again, Kohlberg found individuals developed through a series of stages, from a premoral punishment and obedience orientation to a principled morality and a universal ethical principle orientation.[21] In all these developmental theories, what has happened in the past in the individual's life will always affect the future.

Biologically, the individual also develops, moving from simple reflex responses to the complex control over fine motor movements. Such progressive differentiation is characteristic of the human organism. Specific biological functions such as the menstrual cycle have an ongoing effect on the body. With the onset of puberty, changes in the body structure such as increased breadth of the hips and breast development begin. Such changes persist past the menopause. Although the functioning of the body before puberty and following menopause may

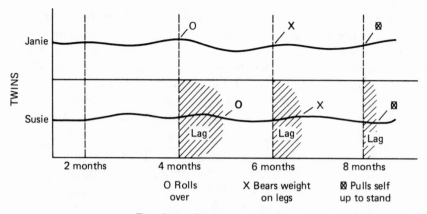

Figure 12-1. Pictorial representation of the developmental lag experienced by one twin, Susie, as a result of leg-casting for six weeks following her two-month birthday.

be said to be similar, the persistence of the identified changes mandates that the postmenopausal functioning be viewed differently from prepuberty functioning, thus illustrating the principle of helicy.

Components of Callista Roy's adaptation model may also be viewed as consistent with Rogers's conceptual framework. Roy's model postulates that the individual's physiologic adaptation, self-concept, role function, and relations with others are the results of interactions with the environment. The environment consists of stimuli, status positions, and persons.[22] The physiological adaptation to the environmental stimulus of altitude change such as that experienced by mountain climbers demonstrates the mutual interaction between the individual and the environment. The simultaneous change in the mountain climber and in the altitude is consistent with the principle of complementarity.

According to Roy, the individual's adaptation of self-concept is affected by the individuals who become part of the environment.[23] Rogers's principle of helicy postulates that each new mutual interaction will promote continuous innovative changes. For example, a woman who is a wife and mother has developed a self-concept that is consistent with her perceptions of her interactions with husband and children. When that same woman then becomes a college student, interactions with faculty, students, and the college environment will promote changes and adaptations in her self-concept.

This mother/wife/student will have a change in her environment and therefore a change in her interaction with that environment. This is representative of complementarity. The new environment of a university will include new faculty, new peers, new books, and new learning experiences in laboratories; and the new environment will cause changes in the old environment—the home—and how the woman interacts with the environment there. At specified points in time the changes caused by the new environment create changes in the life pattern in which she has been functioning.

As the mother/wife/student grows and changes because of her interaction with faculty, peers, and the college environment, she will integrate the material presented and will adapt—emerging from the program as a different woman. This adaptation will affect the old rhythms that have related to her former life style. Before entering the program the mother of the family always cooked the meals; after she enters the program another member of the family may assume the cooking role, thus changing the rhythms of family functioning. Rogers's principle of helicy can be utilized in the changes of rhythms occurring because of the change in the environment.

Resonancy examines the variations occurring during the life process of the "whole" man. The experiences as a student mandate changes in the wife/mother. Because of the progression in space-time, the wife/mother/student can never return to the wife/mother unaffected by the experience of being a student.

USE OF ROGERS'S PRINCIPLES IN THE NURSING PROCESS

If the profession of nursing is concerned with human beings in their wholeness, the principles of homeodynamics would provide guidelines for predicting the nature and direction of the individual's development as responses to health-related problems are made. Using these guidelines, the professional practice of nursing would then seek to promote symphonic interaction between human beings and their environments, to strengthen the coherence and integrity of the human field, and to direct and redirect patterning of the human and environmental fields for the realization of maximum health.[24] These goals would be reflected in the nursing process.

To successfully utilize the principles of homeodynamics, there needs to be a consideration of the nurse and an involvement of both the nurse and the client in the nursing process. If anything or anyone external to the individual is part of the environment, then the nurse would be part of the client's environment. Since the nurse serves as the facilitator of the nursing process, it is vital that she be considered an integral part of the environment. Because of the mutual interaction of the individual and the environment, it is implied that the client is a willing, integral participant in the nursing process. Nursing, then, is working *with* the client, not *to* or *for* the client. This involvement in the nursing process by the nurse demonstrates concern for the total person, rather than one aspect, one problem, or a limited segment of need fulfillment.[25]

In the nursing assessment phase of the nursing process, all facts and opinions about the individual and the environment are collected. Because of our limited measuring devices and data-collection tools, the information collected in the assessment is frequently of an isolate or particulate nature. However, to implement the guidelines, the analysis of the data must be in such a fashion as to reflect wholeness. This may be done by asking several questions and seeking the responses from the collected data.

The first series of questions reflect the principle of complementarity. What is the interaction between man and the environment? How has one adjusted to the other? Are there any maladjustment factors present? Are they able to work together? What factors support or undermine this working relationship? If the individual is in an environment that is not the normal one, how are the two environments different? Based on the differences, what kind of predictions can be made about the individual's interaction with this new environment?

The next series of questions would reflect the principle of resonancy. How has the life process of the individual progressed? What kind of variations have occurred during the course of this life process? What factors have influenced these variations? What role has the environment played in these variations? How would a strange environment affect the individual's life process?

The last series of questions would be influenced by the principle of helicy. What kind of rhythms are reflected in the collected data? How complex are these rhythms? Are they old established rhythms or new emerging ones? How does the environment support these rhythms? If the individual is in a strange environment, how will these rhythms be affected by the new environment? What sequential stages of development has the individual passed through? What were the effects? How has the environment supported or retarded the progress of the individual? How will a new environment affect this progress? What kinds of goals does the individual have? How have these goals affected development? Where do the individuals wish to go as reflected by their goals? What kind of new vistas are sought?

To reflect the idea of patterning, additional questions for the principle of helicy would be considered. What kinds of patterns characterize the individual? How have the patterns developed? What kinds of past experience have influenced the development of specified patterns? How has the environment promoted certain patterns? How complex are the patterns? How has time affected the patterns? Although these questions may be answered, it must be remembered that the responses reflect a specific point in space-time. Consequently, the identified patterns are not static but rather ever-changing, reflecting both a change in time and additional new past experiences.

By no means are these questions all-inclusive, but using them as a reference will help provide the nurse with a view of the whole individual. It will identify individual differences and the sequential cross-sectional patterning in the life process. It will also show the total pattern of events for the person at any given point in space-time.[26] The nursing assessment, then, is an assessment of the whole human being and not an assessment of only physical or mental status. It is an assessment of health and health potential for the individual and not an assessment of an illness or a disease process. As a result, the individual is paramount, not the disease.

As a result of the nursing assessment, a conclusion is drawn about the individual. This conclusion is the nursing diagnosis, the second step in the nursing process, and it will reflect the principles of homeodynamics. Rhythms, patterns, complexity, interactions, and life-process variations would become evident. Such a nursing diagnosis would not be consistent with the problem-oriented medical record system for providing care. In the problem-oriented system, a problem would be identified at this state that should be stated as a symptom, finding, or (medical) diagnosis.[27] As such, the problem would reflect a piece of the individual and not the whole human being. Although also imperfect, the nursing diagnoses developed by Kristine Gebbie and Mary Ann Lavin have a greater potential for usefulness within Rogers's framework because they tend to reflect a more holistic view of the individual.[28]

The purpose of the nursing diagnosis is to provide a framework within which the nursing intervention is planned and implemented. Consequently, the thrust of the nursing intervention will depend on the focus of the nursing diagnosis. The focus on complementarity will require implementation within the environment as well as within the individual. It can be expected that change in one will cause simultaneous change in the other. Because of the individual's interaction with the environment, health problems cannot be separated from the world's social ills. Therefore, these problems cannot be dealt with effectively by means of the commonly accepted transitional, disease-oriented measures.[29] Creativity and imagination become essential.

Resonancy requires that the nursing plan be geared toward supporting or modifying variations in the life process of the whole human being. Because the human life process is a unidirectional phenomenon, the intervention cannot be aimed at returning the individual to a former level of existence; rather, the nurse helps the individual move forward to a higher, more complex level of existence.

Nursing planning in the area of helicy requires an acceptance of individual differences as an expression of evolutionary emergence. The strategies are geared at supporting or modifying rhythms and life goals. To do this requires the informed and active participation of the client in the nursing process. The concept of the unitary human and a recognition of the human being's capacity to feel and to reason will enable the nurse to assist the individual in the resolution of the health problem and in the setting of goals directed toward achieving health.[30] Health will not be achieved by promoting homeostasis and equilibrium, but rather by taking steps to enhance dynamism and complexity within the individual.

Additionally, helicy requires that the nursing plan be geared toward promoting dynamic repatterning of the whole human being. This repatterning includes the individual's relationship to self and to the environment so that the total potential as a human being can be developed. This repatterning is aimed at assisting people to develop patterns of living that coordinate with environmental changes rather than conflict with them.[31] Although the pattern may be altered or maintained, it must be remembered that this is an evolving, ever-changing pattern rather than a static, constant phenomenon.

Regardless of the focus, the aim of the nursing plan is the attainment of an optimum state of health for the individual. This state of health may not be the ideal but will be the maximum health that is potentially possible for the individual.[32] Generally, implementation strategies will seek to strengthen the integrity of the individual-environment relationship and to give direction to humanity's struggle to achieve new levels of well-being. By assisting individuals to mobilize their resources, consciously and unconsciously, their integrity will be heightened.[33]

If attainment of an optimum state of health is the aim of the nursing plan, then it becomes the focus for nursing evaluation, the final phase of the nursing process. Has the integrity of the individual-environment relationship been strengthened? Have resources been mobilized? Has the patterning of the human and environmental fields been directed toward the realization of maximum health potential? Only when the nursing goal of the highest possible health state has been realized can nursing interventions be evaluated as effective.

A schematic representation of the relationship between the principles of homeodynamics and the elements of the nursing process is presented in Table 12-1. As can be seen, there is no absolute distinction between the areas covered by the various principles. Table 12-2 attempts to apply the generalities to the specific situation of Janie who is hospitalized. In no way is either figure designed to be all-inclusive. Rather, they are offered as an attempt to make rather abstract ideas more concrete and operational.

LIMITATIONS OF ROGERS'S
PRINCIPLES OF HOMEODYNAMICS

Although the principles of homeodynamics are consistent with the universally accepted aims and goals of nursing, there are major limitations to the universal implementation of the principles. Many persons will have difficulty understanding the principles. Even though basic assumptions are provided and the principles are defined, the framework remains an abstract phenomenon. Terms have not been sufficiently operationalized to provide for clear understanding.[34] By operationalizing terms is meant the description of a set of physical procedures that must be carried out in order to assign to every case a value for the concept.[35] For example, to operationalize the concept of width is to place a tool consisting of the units of inches or centimeters along the edge of the item to be measured and count the units.

Because of the lack of operational definitions, research done to support or verify the principles provides questionable results. Operational definitions are needed for the development of hypotheses that test the theoretical concepts, and for the selection of tools that will adequately measure the concepts involved.[36] Without such definitions just what was confirmed or not confirmed by these studies is in doubt.[37]

At this stage in the development of nursing science, tools that

Table 12-1

Relationship of the Principles of Homeodynamics to the Nursing Process

Components of the Nursing Process	Principles of Homeodynamics		
	Complementarity	Resonancy	Helicy
Nursing assessment component	Look at interaction of the individual and the environment. How they work together rather than what they are like in isolation.	Look at the variations occurring during the life process of the whole human being.	Look at the rhythmic life patterns of the individual and the environment. Progression of time of necessity creates changes in the rhythmic life patterns of the whole human being. Look at life goals. Be aware of growing complexity of the whole human being.
Nursing diagnosis component	Reflects interaction of the individual and the environmental fields.	Reflects the variations in the life process of the whole individual.	Reflect the rhythmic pattern of the individual and environmental fields.
Nursing plan for implementation component	Intervene in environment as well as in the individual. Change promoted in one area will cause simultaneous change in the other—simultaneous molding.	Support or modify variations in the life process of the whole individual.	Promote dynamic rhythmic repatterning of both the individual and the environment. Accept differences as an expression of evolutionary emergence. Promote dynamism and complexity rather than homeostasis and equilibrium. Support or modify life goals.
Nursing evaluation component	Evaluate changes in the interaction that has occurred.	Evaluate the modification made in the variations of the life process of the whole human being.	Evaluate rhythmic repatterning of the individual and the environment. Evaluate goal-directedness. Evaluate relationship of goal to the whole individual.

Table 12-2

Relationship of the Principles of Homeodynamics to the Nursing Process for Janie

Components of the Nursing Process	Principles of Homeodynamics		
	Complementarity	Resonancy	Helicy
Nursing assessment component	1. How does Janie see her environment? 2. What kind of differences are there between the hospital and her home? 3. How is she reacting to the changes in her environment? 4. How does her health problem and the environment affect each other?	1. What is Janie's past history? 2. What kind of deviations from the expected norms have there been? 3. Were these deviations individually or environmentally related? 4. What is the reason for the hospitalization? 5. How will this affect her life?	1. What are Janie's normal behavior patterns and routine? 2. Were the behaviors or routines undergoing a change prior to her admission? 3. What kinds of activities can she perform? 4. What kinds of past experiences has she had? 5. How might those experiences influence her current situation? 6. What is Janie's developmental level? 7. Will the hospital environment support or retard developmental progress? 8. What are Janie's goals?
Nursing diagnosis component	1. What is the nature of the interaction between Janie and the hospital?	1. What is the interference this hospitalization will make in Janie's life?	1. What are the rhythmic patterns that are being exhibited?

Principles of Homeodynamics

Components of the Nursing Process	Complementarity	Resonancy	Helicy
Nursing plan for implementation component	1. How can the hospital environment be modified to reduce the differences identified? 2. How can Janie be helped to understand the differences that cannot be eliminated? 3. How can her health potential be improved by manipulating the environment?	1. How can Janie's normal development be promoted? 2. How can the effects of the interferences be minimized?	1. How can Janie's normal behavioral patterns and routines be promoted in the hospital? 2. What kind of modifications can be made to promote her normal behavioral patterns and routines? 3. What kind of provisions can be made to promote her normal growth and development? 4. How can Janie be helped to develop successful rhythmic behavioral patterns within the hospital environment? 5. How can Janie be helped to reach her goals?
Nursing evaluation component	1. Has Janie's behavior changed as a result of environmental modification? 2. What kind of new reactions are now taking place?	1. Is Janie developing normally, based on theorists? 2. Has the interference with development been minimized?	1. What kind of rhythmic repatterning has taken place? 2. Is Janie's development being supported? 3. Is she moving toward her goals?

will adequately assess human beings in their totality are nonexistent. Without such tools, the ability to utilize or test the framework successfully is virtually impossible. The inability to adequately utilize or test the framework makes successful nursing implementation difficult. Thus, utilization of principles of homeodynamics in its totality is limited. At best, varying aspects of the principles can be applied to nursing practice in a very limited fashion.

CONCLUSIONS

Despite certain limitations, as discussed in the previous section, the theory and framework do attempt to describe nursing phenomena by suggesting new lines of reasoning and by offering new avenues of exploration. This theory is an attempt to establish structure and meaning for the world of nursing.[38] As such, further development through concretizing definitions and hypothesizing explicit relationships is warranted. Only when this is done can the nursing community begin to truly reap the rewards of the effective utilization of Rogers's conceptual framework.

SUMMARY

Building on a broad theoretical base from a variety of disciplines, Rogers developed the principles of homeodynamics. Inherent in the principles are five basic assumptions: (1) the human being is a unified whole possessing individual integrity and manifesting characteristics that are more than and different from the sum of the parts; (2) the individual and the environment are continuously exchanging matter and energy with each other; (3) life process of human beings evolves irreversibly and unidirectionally along a space-time continuum; (4) pattern and organization identify human beings and reflect their innovative wholeness; and (5) the individual is characterized by the capacity for abstraction and imagery, language and thought, sensation and emotion. The principles of homeodynamics, which include the principles of complementarity, helicy, and resonancy, are compared to general system theory, developmental theories, and adaptation theories. Ways to utilize the principles in the nursing process are explored. The difficulty in understanding the principles, the lack of operational definitions, and inadequate tools for measurement are the major limitations to the effective utilization of this theory.

NOTES

1. Martha E. Rogers, *The Theoretical Basis of Nursing* (Philadelphia: F. A. Davis Co., 1970), pp. vii, ix.
2. Ibid., p. 4.
3. Ibid., p. 10.
4. Ibid., pp. 12–14.
5. Alvin Toffler, *Future Shock* (New York: Bantam Books, 1970), p. 30.
6. Martha E. Rogers, "Accountability," Convention address, University of Utah College of Nursing, June 5, 1971, p. 3.
7. Rogers, *The Theoretical Basis of Nursing*, pp. 47–73.
8. Ludwig von Bertalanffy, *General System Theory* (New York: George Braziller, Inc., 1968), p. 38.
9. Mary Elizabeth Hazzard, "An Overview of Systems Theory," *Nursing Clinics of North America*, 6, no. 3 (September 1971), 385.
10. von Bertalanffy, *General System Theory*, p. 37.
11. Ibid., pp. 27–28.
12. Rogers, *The Theoretical Basis of Nursing*, vii, pp. 84–85.
13. Ibid., pp. 97–102; and idem, "Nursing Science: A Science of Unitary Man," Distinguished Lecture Series, Wright State University, Dayton, Ohio, October 20, 1978.
14. Hazzard, "An Overview of Systems Theory," pp. 389–390.
15. Alvin L. Bertrand, *Social Organization* (Philadelphia: F. A. Davis Co., 1972), p. 99.
16. Hazzard, "An Overview of Systems Theory," p. 390.
17. Erik Erikson, *Childhood and Society*, 2nd ed. (New York: W. W. Norton & Company, Inc., 1963), pp. 247–274.
18. Robert Havinghurst, *Developmental Tasks and Education*, 3rd ed. (New York: David McKay Co., 1972).
19. Jean Piaget and Rachel Inhelder, *The Psychology of the Child* (New York: Basic Books, Inc., 1969).
20. Lawrence Kohlberg, *Collected Papers on Moral Development and Moral Education* (Cambridge, Mass.: Moral Education and Research Foundation, 1973).
21. Ibid.
22. Callista Roy, "The Roy Adaptation Model," in *Conceptual Models for Nursing Practice*, Joan P. Riehl and Callista Roy, eds. (New York: Appleton-Century-Crofts, 1974), p. 138.
23. Ibid., p. 138.

24. Rogers, *The Theoretical Basis of Nursing*, p. 122.
25. Helen Yura and Mary B. Walsh, *The Nursing Process* (New York: Appleton-Century-Crofts, 1973), p. 72.
26. Callista Roy, "Rogers' Theoretical Basis of Nursing," in *Conceptual Models for Nursing Practice*, Joan P. Riehl and Callista Roy, eds. (New York: Appleton-Century-Crofts, 1974), pp. 98–99.
27. Rosemarian Berni and Helen Readey, *Problem-Oriented Medical Record Implementation* (St. Louis, Mo.: The C. V. Mosby Co., 1975).
28. Kristine M. Gebbie and Mary Ann Lavin, eds., *Classification of Nursing Diagnoses* (St. Louis, Mo.: The C. V. Mosby Co., 1975).
29. Rogers, *The Theoretical Basis of Nursing*, p. 134.
30. Ibid.
31. Roy, "Rogers' Theoretical Basis of Nursing," p. 99.
32. Ibid., pp. 97, 99.
33. Rogers, *The Theoretical Basis of Nursing*, pp. 134, 139.
34. Imogene King, *Toward a Theory for Nursing* (New York: John Wiley & Sons, Inc., 1971).
35. Margaret E. Hardy, "Theories: Components, Development, Evaluation," *Nursing Research*, 23, no. 2 (March-April 1974), 101.
36. Ibid., p. 105.
37. Rogers, *The Theoretical Basis of Nursing*, pp. 103–128.
38. Hardy, "Theories: Components, Development, Evaluation," p. 105.

REFERENCES

BERNI, ROSEMARIAN, and HELEN READEY, *Problem-Oriented Medical Record Implementation*. St. Louis, Mo.: The C. V. Mosby Co., 1974.
BERTRAND, ALVIN L., *Social Organization*. Philadelphia: F. A. Davis Co., 1972.
ERIKSON, ERIK, *Childhood and Society*, 2nd ed. New York: W. W. Norton & Company, Inc., 1963.
GEBBIE, KRISTINE M., and MARY ANN LAVIN, eds., *Classification of Nursing Diagnoses*. St. Louis, Mo.: The C. V. Mosby Co., 1975.
HARDY, MARGARET E., "Theories: Components, Development, Evaluation," in *Nursing Research*, 23, no. 2 (March-April 1974), 100–107.
HAVINGHURST, ROBERT, *Developmental Tasks and Education*, 3rd ed. New York: David McKay Co., 1972.
HAZZARD, MARY ELIZABETH, "An Overview of Systems Theory," *Nursing Clinics of North America*, 6, no. 3 (September 1971), 385–393.
KING, IMOGENE, *Toward a Theory for Nursing*, New York: John Wiley & Sons, Inc., 1971.
KOHLBERG, LAWRENCE, *Collected Papers on Moral Development and Moral Education*. Cambridge, Mass.: Moral Education and Research Foundation, 1973.

PIAGET, JEAN, and RACHEL INHELDER, *The Psychology of the Child.* New York: Basic Books, Inc., 1969.

ROGERS, MARTHA E., *The Theoretical Basis of Nursing.* Philadelphia: F. A. Davis Co., 1970.

———, "Accountability," convention address, University of Utah College of Nursing, June 5, 1971.

———, "Nursing Science: A Science of Unitary Man," Distinguished Lecture Series, Wright State University, Dayton, Ohio, October 20, 1978.

ROY, CALLISTA, "Rogers's Theoretical Basis of Nursing," in *Conceptual Models for Nursing Practice,* pp. 96–99, Joan P. Riehl and Callista Roy, eds. New York: Appleton-Century-Crofts, 1974.

———, "The Roy Adaptation Model," in *Conceptual Models for Nursing Practice,* pp. 135–144, Joan P. Riehl and Callista Roy, eds., New York: Appleton-Century-Crofts, 1974.

SAFIER, GWENDOLYN, *Contemporary American Leaders in Nursing.* New York: McGraw-Hill Book Company, 1977.

TOFFLER, ALVIN, *Future Shock.* New York: Bantam Books, 1970.

VON BERTALANFFY, LUDWIG, *General System Theory.* New York: George Braziller, Inc., 1968.

YURA, HELEN, and MARY B. WALSH, *The Nursing Process.* New York: Appleton-Century-Crofts, 1973.

13

IMOGENE M. KING

Julia B. George

Imogene King received her basic nursing education from St. John's Hospital School of Nursing, St. Louis, Missouri. Her Ed.D. is from Teachers College, Columbia University, New York.

King has had experiences in nursing as an administrator, an educator, and a practitioner. Her positions in nursing education have included Director, School of Nursing, The Ohio State University, Columbus, Ohio; and Professor of Nursing, Loyola University of Chicago, Chicago, Illinois.

Imogene M. King's *Toward a Theory for Nursing: General Concepts of Human Behavior* was published in 1971.[1] This book grew from King's thoughts about the vast amounts of knowledge available to nurses and the difficulty this presented to the individual nurse in choosing the facts relevant to a given situation.[2] From the early 1960s the many and rapid advances in science and technology were having a great impact on the profession of nursing as well as on other components of society. Also, as emerging professionals, some nurses were beginning to seek the knowledge base specific to nursing practice and to challenge the existing role of the nurse. Beginning with an historical overview, King identified concepts basic to nursing.

In the preface of her book, King clearly states she is proposing a conceptual framework for nursing and not a nursing theory. As she denotes in the title, her purpose was to help move *toward* a theory for nursing. King says that the essential characteristics of nursing are elements or properties that have continued to exist, function, and influence in spite of the location or environment of nursing.[3] In relation to nursing she discusses the concepts of man, social systems, perceptions, interpersonal relationships, and health. As her extensive documentation indicates, she has drawn from a wide variety of sources in developing these concepts.

KING'S FIVE CONCEPTS

Man

Man, in the universal term as human being, is the central focus of King's framework. Three basic premises of man are proposed. These are: (1) man as a *reacting* being, (2) man as a *time-oriented* being, and (3) man as a *social* being.[4] As a reacting being, man must have an awareness of other persons, things, and events in his environment. At any given time, this awareness leads to a response to the environmental stimuli based on the individual's perceptions, expectations, and needs. This response occurs as a composite of mind and body—man using energy to react as a total organism to experiences and events.

At any particular moment, man's reaction is influenced by time orientation. Each person's present has its base in past experiences. Similarly, awareness of the present shapes a person's ideas of the future. According to Martha Rogers, time cannot be reversed in the life cycle—no one can go back to a previous time in personal history.[5] Developmental theorists, such as Erikson and Piaget, indicate individuals develop over a period of time in specific, orderly phases, each phase dependent on the previous ones.[6] Present reactions are related to developmental phase and past experiences. Man can recall *past* events to influence *present* decisions and can plan to achieve *future* goals based on past and present experiences.

Man also reacts in a given time space as a social being. Man has a continual exchange with persons in the environment. He has language, a symbolic method of communication that facilitates the exchange of explicit thoughts and feelings as well as the description of concrete items and abstract ideas. The factors of interaction and communication enable man to function in social systems.

In addition to the three basic premises, King also discusses seven common characteristics of man.[7] These characteristics, although not all-inclusive, are abilities necessary for the functioning of the three basic premises. First, man has the ability to *perceive*. Each person develops her/his own concepts through personal awareness and inter-pretation of individual and multiple objects, persons, events, or things. These concepts and perceptions influence behavior and, thus, life and health. *Thinking*, the second ability, is based on man's inquiring mind. Perception and thinking allow and help man to generalize, discriminate, and identify relationships. Third is the ability to *feel*, to have emotions about and reaction to the environment—both human and nonhuman. Fourth, man is able to *choose* between alternative courses of action. Obviously, the abilities to perceive and think are inherent in making choices. Choices are also influenced by feelings. Closely associated with thinking and choosing alternatives is the fifth ability—to *set goals*. Sixth, man is able to *select the means to achieve the goals* that have been set. Seventh, and a basis for and dependent on many of the other characteristics, man can *make decisions*.

These premises and characteristics are closely related to adaptation theories. The individual as a reactor adapts. Theodore Mills indicates adaptation involves increasing openness, extending the scope of contacts and obligations beyond current boundaries and being able to alter customs and habits.[8] All of these are responses or reactions. Openness and contacts imply a social setting. The willingness to change—to become more open or alter customs—is rooted in past successes. Callista Roy indicates adaptation occurs with positive re-sponse to internal or external change for the promotion of maximum potential for living.[9] Again, response is reaction. Internal or external change relates to environment and social being.

How the individual adapts will be influenced by past experiences and future plans. For example, John and Larry are both twenty-one years old, single, and college students. Due to a recent increase in tuition, neither has adequate financial resources to enroll for the current term. Both are in a similar situation. They adapt in different ways—John applies for a student loan; Larry accepts a full-time job and temporarily suspends his formal education. The differences come partly from the past—John has a good credit rating due to prompt payment of an automobile loan; Larry has never had a loan and has not established a credit rating. The present also exerts an influence— the only job John can find would barely meet his living expenses;

Larry has a job that will allow him to save toward future college expenses. Finally, future plans enter into the adaptation—John is a first-term senior who has the promise of a good job after graduation; Larry has at least three more years of schooling before receiving his degree. Thus, John applies for the loan because he has had a successful past experience in loan repayment, because he cannot find an adequate job currently, and because in a year's time he can complete degree requirements that will allow him to accept a well-paying position and repay the loan. Larry has had no experience with loans, has a job that can help him eventually earn a degree, and he would need a loan or other financial assistance for at least three years. The adaptation of both John and Larry is based on perception, thinking, decision making, goal setting, alternative selection, and feelings.

King states, "Man functions in social systems through interpersonal relationships in terms of his perceptions which influence his life and his health."[10] In this way she relates the central focus, man, to the other concepts of social systems, perception, interpersonal relationships, and health.

Social Systems

Social systems are made up of individuals.

> Groups of individuals join together in a network or system of social relationships to achieve common goals developed about a system of values with an organized set of practices and the methods to regulate practices and administer the rules. The members of the groups interact according to standards or norms based on a set of roles and status.[11]

Also inherent in such networks are behavior patterns, authority, and age gradation.

Values are broad, nonspecific qualities esteemed by the group.[12] Values may include such ideas as truthfulness, honor, or the worth of human life. Norms, standards, or rules that guide and regulate behavior are set by the social system and are accepted by most of the members of the system.[13] Thus, we are expected to salute or otherwise pay respect to the flag of our country when the national anthem is played. Another example of a norm within a given social system would be, "Don't get pregnant unless you are married," or the former practice among the Eskimos and certain Indian tribes of leaving elderly citizens outside the community boundaries to die alone.

Roles are dyadic relationships with socially prescribed behaviors for a particular situation.[14] The position "nurse" is only one-half of a role. To complete the role you must know what or who forms the other half in order to know the expected behaviors. For instance, a different set of behaviors is required of the nurse in each of these roles: nurse/patient, nurse/doctor, nurse/nurse, nurse/nurse's aide, nurse/member of the patient's family, nurse/member of the community, and nurse/community group. All of the roles in a given position make up a role set.

Status is a group of related roles one occupies within the system.[15] It may also be known as status-position. As a new member in a system, an individual may have a limited number of roles in that system. With increased contact in the system or with demonstration of competencies valued by the system, the roles and the status will increase in complexity. In an intellectual community, such as a university setting, the individual with a doctoral degree will have relatively high status due to the competency implied by the doctoral degree. That same degree would grant fewer roles and a less complex status position in a system that places high value on manual labor.

Behavior patterns are expected ways of performance and will vary according to the place of the individual within the system. For instance, although it is acceptable for a two-year-old to "throw a tantrum," similar behavior in a twenty-two-year old is unacceptable. We also have certain expected behaviors for the chairperson of the group, e.g., to lead the meetings—behaviors that are different from those of the secretary, e.g., to record and publish the minutes.

Authority can be defined as the seat of power, or the individual or group within the system who has the right to make decisions that guide others' actions.[16] The authority may be official, like that granted to the position of an elected or appointed leader, or functional, like that granted by the members of the system to those individual(s) who exert influence through such factors as charisma and knowledge.[17] Official and functional authority may or may not rest with the same person or group.

Also seen in social systems is some degree of age gradation. Within the social system of the family, ages may range from the newborn through grandparents or great-grandparents. The age gradation of an industrial health setting may be from eighteen to sixty-five. The social system of a health care setting will have an age gradation dependent on the specialization of the care givers. A well-child clinic will have a smaller gradation than an ambulatory care center where all age groups may be seen.

Nurses will work with three levels of social systems—individual, group, and society. The individual level is the personal social system with the pertinent related concept of perception. The group level is an interpersonal system that includes the family and is associated with interpersonal relationships. The society level is made up of groups in which the focus is on the concept of health.

Perceptions

Perception is "each individual's representation or image of reality,"[18] each one's view of what is going on in the world. What we see is influenced by what we know, what we look for, and what is familiar to us. The outdoorsman picks up clues to impending weather changes, such as cloud formations or wind changes, which the uninitiated would ignore. The experienced labor and delivery room nurse watches for and recognizes the implications of a widely varying fetal heart rate and rhythm. As a further example, what does Figure 13-1 mean to you?

Figure 13-1.

You may well perceive it is just four marks on the page unless you know it is a square that cannot make ends meet!

The nurse needs to be aware of what the individual's perceptions are—of self, family, and friends; of past and ongoing events and of the nurse. The nurse's perceptions of these must also be clearly identified. The next step is to be aware of where the nurse's and the individual's perceptions match and conflict. Ideally, actions will be based on matching perceptions. At the very least, the nurse's actions should not be in conflict with the individual's perceptions. For example, a woman who believes small babies lead to easy delivery may decide to gain no more than ten pounds during pregnancy; whereas the nurse's perception of a desired weight gain may be two to three times this amount and is in direct conflict with this woman's perceptions. Nutrition teaching based on the nurse's perception is not likely to be well received or followed by this woman during pregnancy, unless the perceptions can be brought closer together.

The nurse who seeks to assist an individual in a way perceived as unnecessary by that person is wasting her time and energy. Also, the nurse may be creating an unwillingness in that individual to seek nursing help in the future! Satisfactory interpersonal relationships will increase awareness of perceptions and will assist in increasing continuity between care giver and client.

Interpersonal Relationships

Interpersonal relationships always involve a minimal group of two. An interpersonal relationship is "the interaction of two or more individuals in . . . time for some purpose or goal."[19] The system is a "group" since two or more people are involved. Interpersonal relationships are purposeful. The purpose may range from achieving a healthy mother and baby at the end of a pregnancy, to optimal rehabilitation of the person injured in an accident, to the peaceful achievement of death. To achieve the purpose the relationship must take place over a period of time. The time period may vary from one short contact to several years, depending on the set goals.

Interpersonal relationships in nursing are based on perception, judgment, action, reaction, interaction, and transaction. Perception was defined earlier as the individual's view of reality. Judgment is based on perception. A value is placed on the event. For example, does this nurse really want to help me? Does this individual really wish my help? Action may be verbal or nonverbal and will involve a sequence of behaviors related to recognition of and efforts to control conditions and events. Reaction involves indicating one's perception and action to another. The nurse reacts to the client and the client to the nurse. Interaction then involves not only the exchange of ideas and feelings but also one person doing something for another. Transaction occurs only when both nurse and client are actively working toward a mutually set goal (see Figure 13-2).[20] Action and reaction are basically mental processes on an individual basis. Interaction and transaction are observable group behaviors that include the goal outcome.

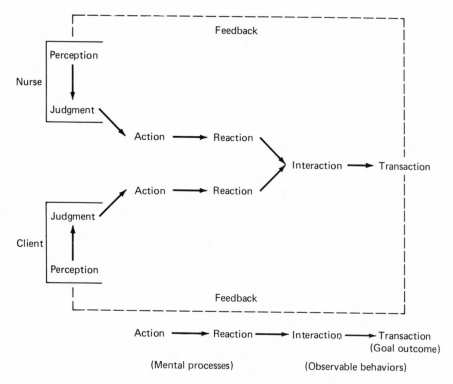

Figure 13-2. Interpersonal relations. [*Adapted from* Imogene M. King, *Toward a Theory of Nursing: General Concepts of Human Behavior* (New York: John Wiley & Sons, Inc., 1971), pp. 26, 92. Used with permission.]

Any nursing involvement with a client will reach the stage of interaction. There will always be an exchange of ideas and/or feelings. The individual who is unable to communicate verbally can communicate feelings through facial expressions and body movements.

Since transaction requires the active involvement of both parties in achieving a mutually set goal, it is not always achievable. Some clients will not be able to participate in the process. For instance, the individual who has a loss of motor function may be unable to participate in active range of motion exercises. The nurse would be interacting with the individual in doing passive range of motion exercises, but transaction would not have been reached due to the client's inability to participate actively.

Interpersonal relationships as discussed by King relate closely to Hildegard Peplau's interpersonal process.[21] Both depend on an exchange between nurse and client and are based on working toward a common goal. A goal of interpersonal relationships will be related to health.

Health

> Health is a dynamic state in the life cycle of an organism that implies continuous adaptation to stresses in the internal and external environment through optimum use of one's resources to achieve maximum potential for daily living.[22]

King's definition of health indicates it is dynamic—an ever-changing process that is a state of being, not a point to be achieved, that is, an ongoing fluid existence rather than a static state. This dynamic state occurs in the life cycle—from conception to death. It is not a consideration for only one age group nor is it limited to any specific point in time. All of society is involved; for a society to have health, it must be at least partially composed of healthy individuals. The individual is continually adapting or using energy to change to meet the requirements of the internal and/or external environment. For the individual, the internal environment consists of the organ systems, cells, hormones, and inner thought processes, in all their intricate and unique interactions. The external environment consists of all things that impact on the person from the outside—air, sound, pollutants, food, other people, animals, machinery.

Stresses are referred to in Hans Selye's terms as demands or calls for action in any sphere—physical, emotional, spiritual, or mental.[23] These may be positive demands and are necessary for living. It is generally accepted that a certain level of tension is necessary to hold our bodies upright, to move a muscle, or to learn. It is only when the demands exceed the organism's ability to adapt that the stress may be considered negative. Resources are anything that the organism can utilize—money, food, friends, knowledge, religious beliefs, values. Also implied in optimum use and maximum potential is the thought that individuals should make the best use of what they have to do the most they can. This is an individual phenomenon as each person has slightly different resources from any other, and each will have a different maximum potential from any other. If illness is considered a deviation from normal, it can be considered a characteristic of health. The deviation may occur as a biological imbalance, an alteration in psychological makeup, or a social conflict.[24]

Nursing

If man is the central focus for social systems, perception, interpersonal relationships, and health, what is *nursing*?

> Nursing is a process of action, reaction, interaction, and transaction whereby nurses assist individuals of any age and socio-economic group to meet their basic needs in performing activities of daily living and to cope with health and illness at some particular point in the life cycle.[25]

In this definition King combines the concepts she has discussed to support nursing as a process involved with social systems, using perception and interpersonal relationships to focus on health. According to the definition of theory as a group of interrelated concepts, this is King's theory statement about nursing.

The process is the basic interpersonal relationship of action, reaction, interaction, and transaction. The social system may be an individual, a group, or a society. King carefully points out that the social system is not limited by age, finances, or social status. The focus of nursing is assisting people to meet basic needs and to perform those activities pertinent to everyday life such as eating, sleeping, communicating with others, donning clothing, or breathing. Also, the nurse is to help a social system at a particular point to face and handle the stresses related to achieving the dynamic state of health for that system.

The nursing process discussed by King is the action, reaction, interaction, transaction chain. However, each of her concepts can be utilized in the nursing process as discussed in Chapter 2.

COMPARISON OF KING'S THEORY AND THE NURSING PROCESS

In *assessment* the nurse acts, reacts, and interacts with people. The perception involved in action and reaction must be considered—both the nurse's view and the client's view—in deciding what data are most pertinent and what analysis should be derived from the data. For example, the mother who is deeply concerned about her child's eating patterns will wish to focus on data related to nutrition rather than discussing family health history.

The nurse seeks to understand the social system of the client. The social systems of the client and the nurse will have an impact on their perceptions. The nurse and the client are more likely to share similar perceptions if they share similar social systems. As the differences in their social systems increase, so will the differences in their perceptions of events. Interpersonal relationships are the basis of the interaction between nurse and client. Without them data collection and analysis would be nearly impossible. The client's health status is the focus of the assessment phase. The nurse is seeking data to discover the client's ability to adapt to stresses, to use resources, and to achieve potential for daily living.

The *nursing diagnosis* is based on the nurse's understanding and analysis of the data about the client's social system, perceptions, interpersonal relationships, and health. The nurse needs knowledge of the client's self-expectations and others' expectations of the client to understand the client's perceptions and adaptation level. For example, pica (perverted appetite) in pregnancy may be extremely detrimental to the health status of both the mother and the fetus. Pica may also be a part of the cultural expectations of the mother. Data are needed as to what unusual substance is being ingested, the extent to which it is being ingested, the extent to which it replaces the desired nutritional intake, and the cultural and emotional implications of the substance to the mother. Analysis of data indicating a pregnant woman is eating five pounds of flour daily, and little else, would lead to the conclusion that she and her baby are in danger. Some nutritional changes are needed, no matter how important the flour ingestion is culturally. In contrast, the woman who is ingesting a small amount of clay, in addition to a well-balanced diet, and who has an adequate hemoglobin level, would be analyzed as functioning at a healthy level and meeting her physical and emotional/cultural needs. The nursing diagnosis would be different in these two situations even though both women could be defined as having pica. In the first instance, the nursing diagnosis could be, "Inadequate nutrition related to pica intake resulting in high-risk pregnancy." In the second case, the nursing diagnosis could be, "Adequate nutrition related to balanced dietary intake and small amount of pica ingestion resulting in normal prenatal development."

In the *planning* and *implementation* phases, ideally transaction will be reached. Planning should involve the setting of mutual goals to move an individual (family, group) toward health in the social system. Also included in planning is discussion of how to reach these goals together, that is, what the nurse can do to assist the individual (family, group) in seeking to reach the goal(s). Again, interpersonal relationships will be a key in these steps. If the nurse and client are not communicating clearly, goals will not be mutually set. Implementation will not achieve transaction and may not result in movement toward mutual goals. The client's social system, values, perceptions, and health status will continue to influence the selection of goals, setting of priorities, and selection of tasks to reach the goals.

In situations where transaction is impossible, planning and implementation may still successfully occur at the interaction level. For example, the individual who cannot exercise active muscle control may be receiving passive range of motion exercises. If this individual also cannot communicate verbally, mutual goal setting is hampered. Since the range of motion exercises are passive, the individual is not actively involved in this implementation. Although the client may have agreed to the goal of maintaining limb mobility, the impaired communication prevents the nurse from knowing the goal is mutual. Without mutual goal setting and active participation of nurse and client in working toward the goal, transaction has not occurred. However, interaction is taking place in the planning and implementation of the exercise.

Again, *evaluation* involves all the concepts. Perceptions of changes are necessary to see movement toward goals. The values from the social system will influence these perceptions. For example, the woman who is a member of a social system that places a high value on starch eating is not likely to perceive a marked decrease in starch intake as positive. The changes may also involve interpersonal relationships between the client and others than the nurse. The client's perceptions will be of utmost importance in evaluating the effect of the changes in this area. Since health is involved in the goals, evaluation includes the data about the client's movement on the health continuum.

The central focus of the conceptual framework and of the nursing process is man. Man is the client. The concepts of social systems, perception, interpersonal relationships, and health all impact on nursing and are important in each phase of the nursing process.

LIMITATIONS OF KING'S THEORY

King does include the four major concepts presented in Chapter 1— man, health, society (social systems), and nursing. She also uses the concept of interpersonal relationships to interrelate man, health, and society for a theory of nursing.

Her theory statement about nursing does not clearly indicate the relationship to society. The statement indicates nurses help individuals. Nursing relationships with groups or society must be inferred from the plural use of individuals and the mention of age and socio-economic group. Support of the concept of groups and society is strong in the book but is not as apparent in the theory statement.

A potentially confusing portion of King's work is her definition of the process of nursing. She identifies the action, reaction, interaction, transaction chain as the process of nursing. The terminology of process of nursing is similar to the nursing process (assess, nursing diagnosis, plan, implement, and evaluate). King's process of nursing is important for carrying out the activities of the nursing process, but it is not as inclusive as the nursing process in Chapter 2. The terms must be used carefully and must be identified clearly to avoid confusion.

Also, in defining nursing King uses the base term *nurse*. Using a word from the same base in a definition weakens the definition. It would be expected that nursing would be done by nurses just as you would expect teaching to be done by teachers!

CONCLUSION

Although King's stated purpose was to present a conceptual framework, she has presented a theory of nursing. Despite the limitations, this theory is applicable to nursing practice. Nurses can, and do, use perceptions and interpersonal relationships to assist clients to work toward health. Since a system can be defined at the level desired, the theory statement would be more inclusive if it were reworded to state that nursing is a process in which a system (individual, group, or society) is assisted.

SUMMARY

In a well-documented manner, King discusses man as the central focus for her concepts of social systems, perceptions, interpersonal relationships, and health. These concepts are interrelated to create a theory statement for nursing.

The use of these concepts in the nursing process is discussed, and examples are given. The major limitations of this theory are the lack of emphasis on social systems in the theory statement and the potential confusion between King's process of nursing and the nursing process.

NOTES

1. Imogene M. King, *Toward a Theory of Nursing: General Concepts of Human Behavior* (New York: John Wiley & Sons, Inc., 1971).
2. Ibid., p. x.
3. Ibid., pp. x, 1–2.
4. Ibid., pp. 87–88.
5. Martha E. Rogers, *An Introduction to the Theoretical Basis of Nursing* (Philadelphia: F. A. Davis Co., 1970), p. 59.
6. Erik Erikson, *Childhood and Society.* 2nd ed. (New York: W. W. Norton & Company, Inc. 1963); and Jean Piaget and Rachel Inhelder, *The Psychology of the Child* (New York: Basic Books, Inc., 1969).
7. King, *Toward a Theory of Nursing*, p. 88.
8. Theodore M. Mills, *The Sociology of Small Groups* (Englewood Cliffs, N.J.: Prentice-Hall, Inc., 1967), p. 21.
9. Sr. Callista Roy, *Introduction to Nursing: An Adaptation Model* (Englewood Cliffs, N.J.: Prentice-Hall, Inc., 1976), p. 11.
10. King, *Toward a Theory of Nursing*, p. 22.
11. Ibid.
12. Alvin L. Bertrand, *Social Organization: A General Systems and Role Theory Perspective* (Philadelphia: F. A. Davis Co., 1972), p. 66.
13. I. Eugene Haas, *Role Conception and Group Consensus* (Columbus, Ohio: Bureau of Business Research, 1963), p. 2.
14. Ibid.
15. Bertrand, *Social Organization*, p. 35.
16. Karen E. Claus and June T. Bailey, *Power and Influence in Health Care* (St. Louis, Mo.: The C. V. Mosby Co., 1977), p. 11.
17. Ibid.
18. King, *Toward a Theory of Nursing*, p. 22.
19. Ibid., p. 23.
20. Ibid., p. 91.
21. Hildegard E. Peplau, *Interpersonal Relations in Nursing* (New York: G. P. Putnam's Sons, 1952).
22. King, *Toward a Theory of Nursing*, p. 24.
23. Hans Selye, *Stress Without Distress* (New York: The New American Library, Inc., 1974), p. 14.
24. King, *Toward a Theory of Nursing*, p. 70.
25. Ibid., p. 25.

REFERENCES

DAUBENMIRE, M. J., and I. M. KING, "Nursing Process Model: A Systems Approach," *Nursing Outlook*, August 1973, pp. 512–517.

KING, IMOGENE M., "A Conceptual Frame of Reference for Nursing," *Nursing Research*, January-February 1968, pp. 27–31.

————, "The Health Care System: Nursing Intervention Subsystem," in W. H. Werley et al., eds. *Health Research: The Systems Approach.* New York: Springer Publishing Co., 1976.

————, "Nursing Theory-Problem and Prospect," *Nursing Science*, October 1964, pp. 394–403.

————, "Planning for Change," *Ohio Nurses Review*, August 1970, pp. 4–7.

14

SISTER CALLISTA ROY

Julia Gallagher Galbreath

Sister Callista Roy (1939–   ) is the Chairman of the Depart-
ment of Nursing at Mount Saint Mary's College in Los Angeles.
She is a fellow of the American Academy of Nursing and a
member of Sigma Theta Tau. Unfolding of the Roy adaptation
model as a conceptual framework for nursing began during her
graduate study at the University of California in 1964. Roy credits
Dorothy E. Johnson as having a strong influence in stimulating
her creative processes. In 1968, fellow faculty at Mount Saint
Mary's College voted unanimously to adopt the adaptation frame-
work as the philosophical basis of the nursing curriculum. Roy,
again, credits Johnson for encouraging her to publish her work.
Resulting publications include Introduction to Nursing: An
Adaptation Model.[1] *Roy has presented many lectures and work-*
shops focusing on the conceptual model of nursing based on
adaptation. She has also given her attention to the development of
nursing taxonomy and nursing diagnosis by active participation in
the regional conferences on classification of nursing diagnosis. Fi-
nally, Roy is committed to the researching of the elements of her
model and has completed clinical research in this area and prom-
ises more research study in the future.

There are three major elements of Roy's adaptation model. First, Roy develops her concept of *man*—the client and the recipient of nursing care. Second, Roy's model represents the goal of nursing, which is to promote *adaptation* through adaptive modes. Finally, the model maps the *process of nursing activities*, most significant of which are nursing assessment of client behaviors and nursing interventions.

CONCEPT—MAN

Roy's model of nursing practice is based on her philosophy of man. She considers man a biopsychosocial being, who, to be properly understood, must be considered as a unit or a whole.[2] The holistic nature of man has been supported by other nursing theorists including Martha Rogers.[3] General systems theory, too, supports the concept of holism. A whole is different from and more than the summation of its individual parts. Hence, the individual is more than one part plus another part. He is an integrated system whose parts have relationships among them. The professional nurse must be interested in the total human being, not just one particular part.

Man-Environment Interaction

Basic to the Roy model is the belief that man is in constant interaction with his environment.[4] Since man is a living system, he requires matter, energy, and information from his environment. In general systems theory this characteristic of a living system is called *openness*. Halbert Dunn calls our attention to the smallest unit of life, the cell. The cell is a living, open system. The cell has its inner and outer worlds. From its outer world it must draw forth the substances it needs to survive. Within itself the cell must maintain order over its vast numbers of molecules.[5] These system qualities are, also, held by man. The constant interaction of man with his environment is characterized by both internal and external change. Within this changing world, man must maintain the integrity of himself; that is, he must adapt.

Adaptation

Roy states that man copes with environmental change through biopsychosocial adaptive mechanisms.[6] Some adaptive mechanisms are inherited or genetic processes, such as the white blood cell defense system against bacteria seeking to invade the body. Other mechanisms are learned, such as the use of antiseptics to cleanse a wound. Since change characterizes our internal and external worlds, one might say that the human capacity to adapt is great. However, it is not without its limits. The process of adaptation occurs when the individual positively responds to internal or external change. One's maximum potential for living relates to health. Health is a state of human functioning whereby the person continually adapts to change. According to Roy, health can be viewed along a continuum that flows from death and extreme poor health, through poor health, to a midpoint of normal health. The health continuum moves from this midpoint to good health, to high-level wellness, to peak health (see Figure 14-1).[7]

Death	Extremely poor health	Poor health	Normal health	Good health	High-level wellness	Peak wellness

Figure 14-1. Roy's health-illness continuum. (Callista Roy, *Introduction to Nursing: An Adaptation Model*, p. 11 © 1976. Used with permission of Prentice-Hall, Inc., Englewood Cliffs, New Jersey.)

Adaptation Level

What factors are significant in determining whether an individual will be capable of adapting to the change occurring in the internal or external worlds? Roy cites Harry Helson in identifying two factors:

1. The degree of environmental change.
2. The state of the person's coping.[8]

Examples of environmental change include snow, temperature change, presence of a virus, radiation from a nuclear explosion, and industrial pollution. Alvin Toffler's book *Future Shock* focuses on the concept of rapid change in the environment of modern society and the adaptive response that is necessary to cope with these changes.[9] Environmental change interfaces with the individual's state of coping, the other significant element in adaptation to change. The condition of the person or his state of coping is his *adaptation level*. The individual's adaptation level will determine whether a positive response to internal or external environmental change will be elicited. The individual's adaptation level is determined by the *focal*, *contextual*, and *residual* stimuli. In any environment-human interaction, the environmental change is the *focal stimulus*. *Contextual stimuli* are all other stimuli of the person's internal or external world that influence the situation and are measurable or reported by the person. *Residual stimuli* are the "makeup" or characteristics of the individual that are present and relevant to the situation but are more elusive or difficult to measure objectively.[10] Consider the following situation.

Example. A thirty-two-year-old woman and her daughter go to a closed garage where a car has been parked with its engine running. The child becomes dizzy and the mother has to carry her out of the garage.

The running motor of a car in the closed garage significantly alters the gaseous composition of the air. The *focal stimulus* would be the presence of carbon monoxide in the garage. Significant *contextual stimuli* would include the size, age, vital lung capacity of the individuals, as well as the outside temperature, the presence of windows in the garage, time spent in the garage, and all other stimuli present. *Residual stimuli* would include the mother's past experience with emergencies, the child's history of asthma, and any other residual characteristics that might influence the situation.

If the individual's adaptation level is viewed as a line, the zone of adaptation is the distance above and below the line that indicates the limit of individual adaptation capacity. When the total stimuli—focal, contextual, and residual—fall within the individual's zone of adaptation, a positive response to change is made. The positive response to change is called *adaptation*. However, when the total stimuli fall outside the individual's zone of adaptation, a negative response results. In other words, maladaptation occurs. Roy depicts the individual's zone of adaptation and relates this to the adaptation level and the response to the stimuli (see Figure 14-2).[11]

In our example, the mother's adaptation level, that is, the total focal, contextual, and residual stimuli, fell within the woman's zone of adaptation, and a positive adaptive response was made. The mother was able to walk out of the garage, carrying her child in her arms. However, for the child the total stimuli fell outside her adaptation zone and a negative outcome resulted. The child became dizzy and put her head down in an attempt to nap. If her mother had not carried her out of the garage, her physiological integrity would have been threatened.

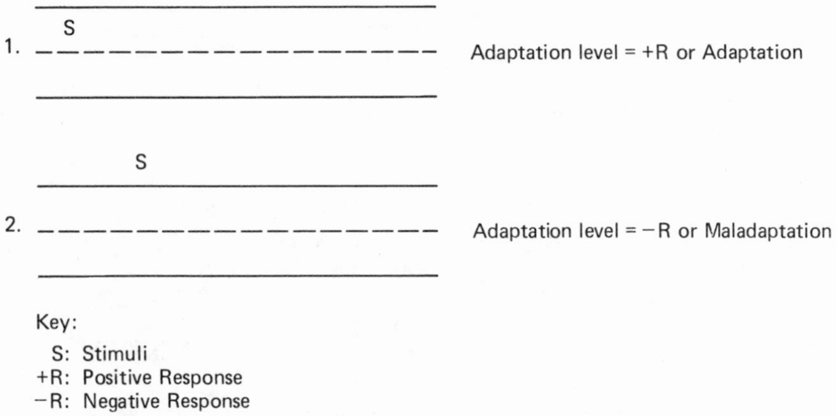

Figure 14-2. Helson's zone of adaptation. (Callista Roy, *Introduction to Nursing: An Adaptation Model,* p. 13, © 1976. Used with permission of Prentice-Hall, Inc., Englewood Cliffs, New Jersey.)

MODES OF ADAPTATION

Roy identifies four distinct modes or ways of adapting by which man responds to change: (1) physiological needs, (2) self-concept, (3) role function, and (4) interdependence. Adaptive modes are activated when need excesses or deficits are created within the individual.[12] The concept of needs has been given much attention by social scientists. Imogene King defines a need as "a state of energy exchange within and external to the organism which leads to behavior."[13] René Dubos sees needs as socially conditioned and not essentially the same from person to person.[14] Roy takes the position that biopsychosocial integrity is the basic need of man. Need deficits or excesses stimulate behavior geared at coping with environmental change.[15]

Physiological Needs Mode

Table 14-1 demonstrates the relationship Roy draws between adaptive modes and related needs. Each mode relates to underlying needs. The physiological adaptive mode relates to the need for physiological integrity. This need is further subdivided into exercise and rest, nutrition and elimination, fluid and electrolytes, oxygen and circulation, regulation of temperature, regulation of senses, and regulation of

Table 14-1

Biopsychosocial Integrity and Adaptive Modes

Need	Adaptive Mode
Physiological integrity	Physiological needs: exercise and rest nutrition and elimination fluids and electrolytes oxygen and circulation regulation of temperature regulation of senses regulation of the endocrine systems
Psychological integrity	Self-concept
Social integrity	Role function
	Interdependence

the endocrine systems. Adaptation occurs as the individual maintains his integrity through positive response to need deficits or excesses.[16]

Many scientists have attempted to identify and categorize basic human physiological needs. Dunn identifies the need for nutrition and elimination of waste and the need for open senses.[17] King identifies the need for comfort, hygiene, safety, rest, exercise, and nutrition.[18] For Roy, however, rest, sleep, exercise, etc., are modes of promoting the satisfaction of the need for physiological integrity. She calls the adaptive modes the *intervening variable* between basic needs and behavior. Adaptation problems occur when behavioral responses to need deficits or excesses are inadequate.[19] Examples of a common adaptation problem related to the need for physiological integrity are dehydration and overhydration.

The mother in the preceding example notices that the cheeks of her daughter become rosy-red and her movements uncoordinated. The mother, too, feels an internal sensation that she cannot identify, and she immediately senses danger. She has sensed that the physiological safety of her daughter, and possibly of herself, is being threatened. A need deficit is created, and the mother's physiological adaptive mode is activated. Her autonomic nervous system takes over, her heart begins to pump blood more rapidly, her mental focus narrows. The autonomic response, often termed the "fight or flight" response, is identified by Roy as the *regulator mechanism*, a key adaptive mechanism. The second key adaptive mechanism is the *cognator mechanism*.[20] The mother in the example utilizes this mechanism as she compares the stimuli of the situation with her previous experience, searching for the cause of the sensation she is feeling and the behaviors of her daughter. She checks her daughter's mouth for a foreign object and thinks quickly if the child might have ingested some type of poison. The word *poison* clicks in her mind, and she looks to see if the garage window is open. The closed window confirms her suspicion that the garage has filled with poison gas. The cognator adaptive mechanism continues to function as she turns off the motor, carries her child out of the garage, and goes to her neighbor's house for help. The threat of losing her child jeopardizes her psychological integrity and creates another need deficit. Her neighbor finds her in a state of shock and bewilderment immediately following the incident.

As our example illustrates, need deficits can be created in more than one area concurrently, and more than one adaptive mode may be activated.

Self-Concept Mode

Roy states that the psychological integrity of the individual is an inner requirement or need. This view is likened to Talcott Parsons's view of the human personality as a system. As such, the personality system has the need to maintain its integrity, which Parsons identifies as system adaptation, goal attainment, integration, and pattern-maintenance.[21]

Operating from Roy's model, Marie Driever has developed the self-concept mode. Driever divides the self-concept into physical self and personal self. She further divides the personal self into the moral-ethical self, self-consistency, self-ideal, and self-esteem. Driever's work is based on theories of self developed primarily by Arthur Coombs and Donald Snygg.[22] Common adaptation problems related to the physical self include loss, such as was evident in our example. Recall the mother's immediate reaction of shock and bewilderment after removing herself and her child from the life-threatening situation. As soon as the reality of the threatened loss become clearer to the mother, Driever predicts that anguish and pain would move into her awareness, and crying would be a predictable response.[23]

Role Function Mode

C. H. Anderson states that regular involvement of man with his fellow is a prerequisite to being fully human.[24] One's concept of oneself, too, is defined by interaction with others. One-to-one interaction between individuals is characterized by the use of both verbal and nonverbal symbolic communication. Interpersonal interaction satisfies the human's need to identify the self in relation to others.[25] Paul Watzlavick concludes that through role interaction the concept of self is confirmed, rejected, or disconfirmed; that is, one's definition of self that underlies one's behaviors can be accepted, rejected, or ignored by others. The response of others to the self shapes and reshapes one's behavior.[26] Social interaction occurs within the contexts of family, groups, community, and society.

Jay Haley goes on to say that not all behaviors will be tolerated by people in prolonged contact with one another. Rules of behavior, or one could say *limits of behavior*, will be set that guide one's actions.[27] Behavioral rules or limits that are common within a society are called *norms*. Every person is likely to hold a number of positions. For example, mother, buyer, entertainer, and student are all positions in society. Roy recognizes two elements of role as (1) holding a position in society and (2) interacting with an individual who also holds a position in society. To maintain his social integrity the individual must have others in the environment to interact with, cues of appropriate behavior, and access to the facilities of role performance. When these elements are lacking, need deficits are created, and the role function adaptive mode is activated.[28] A common role function adaptation problem is role conflict.

Interdependence Mode

Social integrity for an individual requires more than just the proper performance of roles in social situations. The individual acts in ways that will result in satisfying his needs for love and support. Through interdependence, one's life gains meaning and purpose. Interdependence is a balance between dependence and independence. Joyce von Landingham is credited by Roy as first developing the idea of interdependence needs.[29] Walter Kempler develops a complementary concept when discussing the human need for separation and unity. Kempler contends that a higher order of unity occurs between significant people when differentiation and separation are allowed.[30] A problem relationship of being overconnected is explored by Ivan Boszormenyi-Nagy. The need of a parent, for example, to keep a child in union with him inhibits his ability to allow separation. The child then becomes the object of the parent's need for self-fulfillment. The implicit danger of the captive role is exploitation.[31] Other common adaptation problems include aggression and loneliness.

NURSING ACTIVITIES
AND THE NURSING PROCESS

How does the nurse determine whether the individual is experiencing an adaptation problem or is adapting but is in need of additional support? Roy suggests that regulator and cognator effectiveness are required so that adaptation can occur, as these are the individual's key adaptive mechanisms. When the nurse observes the failure of either or both of these mechanisms, then maladaptation is suspected.[32]

The nurse, in her *first-level assessment*, observes for signs of autonomic activity, signs that invariably are present when the individual's biopsychosocial integrity is threatened. For example, dehydration can threaten the biological survival of a young child. As less fluid is available for circulation, the child's supply of oxygen to body tissue is compromised. The regulator mechanism responds and the heart rate increases in an effort to meet the body's demands. The nurse must be aware of the body's normal physiological behavior and the signs of autonomic nervous system response. The nurse must, also, be aware of the behavior of the cognator mechanism, reflective of the higher level central nervous system. Here, memory and judgment are conducted by nerve cells. Cognator failure is more difficult to objectively measure. Roy states that cognator ineffectiveness is indicated by:

1. Lack of awareness of the need state.
2. Inability to identify the goal object.
3. Inability to select means to an identified end.
4. Failure to reach a goal object.[33]

The nurse requires a sound knowledge base to understand the behavioral manifestation of coping with change in each of the adaptive modes. With a strong base of scientific knowledge, the nurse makes judgments of client adaptation or maladaptation. The nurse makes these judgments mutually with the client. Often, Roy states, the client is the first to be aware of a coping failure.[34]

Maladaptive behavior, as well as adaptive behavior requiring support, becomes the focus of the nurse. In these identified areas a *second-level assessment* is done by the nurse to identify the focal, contextual, and residual stimuli that combine to determine the individual's adaptation level. It is of critical importance for the nurse to understand the focal, contextual, and residual stimuli present because the nurse's actions will be directed at altering these stimuli so that they will fall within the individual's adaptive zone. The second-level assessment leads the nurse to identification of the adaptation problem.[35] This point of the nursing process is frequently referred to as the *nursing diagnosis*. Appropriate nursing interventions are developed with the goal of changing client behavior.

Intervention is the key nursing activity. Nightingale proposed nursing interventions that manipulated the environment, such as hygiene, fresh air, and sanitation, to create a context that permits healing body mechanisms to function.[36] Roy develops nursing interventions as attempts to manipulate the environment by removing, increasing, decreasing, and/or altering stimuli. The resultant client behavior should be adaptive, promoting movement toward peak health and meeting the individual's needs of biological, social, and psychological integrity.[37] The nurse concludes the nursing process with an *evaluation* of the effectiveness of the nursing intervention in client goal achievement.[38]

Table 14-2 presents an example of the process the nurse follows in assessment and intervention of an adaptation problem. The child in this example is three months old. The regulator mechanism of the child is stimulated by decreased body fluids, and circulation and oxygenation stress create physiological need deficits. The nurse makes a first-level assessment and from the data suspects regulator ineffectiveness. She then directs her attention to the problem area, identifying the focal, contextual, and residual stimuli present. Because the total stimuli fall outside the child's zone of adaptation, a nursing diagnosis is made. Since the nurse has detailed the stimuli related to the adaptation problem, interventions are planned to manipulate these stimuli. The nurse then evaluates the effectiveness of the intervention.

STRENGTHS AND WEAKNESSES
OF ROY'S MODEL

A discussion of Roy's model would not be complete without consideration of its strengths and weaknesses. A major strength of the model is that it guides the nurse to utilize observation and interviewing skills in doing an individualized assessment of each client. Behavior related to the four adaptive modes is collected during the first-level assessment. In considering all the adaptive modes—physiological needs, self-concept, role function, and interdependence—the nurse is likely to have broadened her view of the client.

Additionally, the close association between intervention strategies

Table 14-2

Nursing Process—Adaptation Problem Threatening Physiological Integrity

First-Level Assessment	Second-Level Assessment	Nursing Diagnosis	Nursing Implementation	Evaluation
Increased autonomic nervous system activity	*Focal stimuli*	Intracellular and extracellular fluid deficit due to low oral intake, emesis, and insensible water loss threatening physiological integrity.	30 oz feedings, electrolyte balanced sugar water each hour.	Oral intake 720 cc in 24 hr
Respirations: 45–60/min	Gastrointestinal flu with frequent emesis.			
Pulse: 180–190	*Contextual stimuli*		Have mother feed baby.	Mother with child and fed 10 times a day.
Urine output: 160cc in 8 hr	Age: 3 months			
Crying almost constantly	Weight: 7 lb		Use premature baby nipple to decrease sucking demand.	
	Weight loss: 1 lb, 3 oz in 2 days			
Nursing judgment	Emesis: 200 cc/24 hr			
Regulator ineffectiveness in physiological adaptive mode.	Oral intake: 300 cc/24 hr		Keep blankets off baby when temperature greater than 99°F.	Temperature range: 99–100°F
	Intravenous therapy:			
Physiological needs	(a) 60 cc/hr		Use cool mist room humidifier.	
Oxygen and circulation	(b) 1500 cc/25 hr			
	Urine output: 390 cc/24 hr		Apply hypoallergenic lotion over entire body to decrease skin dryness.	Skin condition—normal turgor
	Temperature: 100.6°F			
	Room temperature: 72°F			All client goals met.
	Room ventilation: poor			
	Long periods of crying			
	Mother absent			
	Lungs: clear			
	Skin: dry, decreased turgor			
	Residual stimuli			
	Premature infant			
	Poor sucking			

and assessment data may clarify for the nurse the importance of individualized assessment of each client. This behavior could replace a common behavior of routinely applying an intervention strategy to a "problem" without consideration of individual variables. For example, routine administration of a sleeping medication for all clients under the nurse's care who are experiencing sleeplessness would not occur if the nurse utilizes this model to guide her behavior. Instead, the nurse would consider each client individually, assess the stimuli impinging on the client, and act to alter the particular stimuli involved. Interventions would then vary relative to individual variables.

The model also suggests that after assessment, the nurse is to make judgments regarding the client's adaptation through the four adaptive modes in relation to need excesses or deficits that are created secondary to environmental change. Recall that need excesses or deficits arise when physiologic integrity, psychic integrity, or social integrity are threatened. Roy fails, however, to define or operationalize these concepts. Without knowing the nature of these phenomena, the nurse is unguided in determining if behavior observed, relating to each adaptive mode, is promoting the underlying integrity of the individual. Is social integrity, for example, the same for all individuals or does it vary relative to time and place? How does the nurse evaluate the effectiveness of nursing interventions without knowing the nature of the goal of her interventions?

One might, also, question the association that is drawn between need deficits or excesses created by a threat to integrity and the behavioral manifestation of that need in the parallel adaptive mode (review Table 14-1). The model suggests that need deficits or excesses related to a threat to physiological integrity would be manifested primarily by behavior in the self-concept adaptive mode. Might the behavioral manifestation of a need deficit related to the loss of a loved object, for example, just as likely be manifested in the physiological needs mode by the behavior of overeating? And, since need deficits or excesses are not directly observable, how can the nurse be sure that observed behavior related to an adaptive mode represents a need deficit identified by the model as parallel to the mode? The basic underlying question evolves around the major assumption of the model that man is a biopsychosocial being by nature. Does such a conceptualization of an individual perceive his wholeness and integrity? Does this conceptual approach truly reflect the nature of man's relationship with his environment? Only further research of the model can give us this answer.

SUMMARY

The Roy adaptation model presents a framework for the professional practice of nursing. Man is viewed as a whole being, in constant interaction with his environment, one who adapts to change through four adaptive modes. The four modes are physiological needs, self-concept, role function, and interdependence. Activation of these modes occurs when need deficits or excesses are created secondary to the environmental change. The regulator and cognator mechanisms reflect respectively the autonomic and central nervous systems. The presence of regulator or cognator mechanism ineffectiveness signals maladaptation. The nurse assesses the human as a whole by considering objective and subjective data related to each adaptive mode. Nurse and client mutually identify regulator or cognator ineffectiveness. With areas of focus thus decided, the nurse identifies the focal, contextual, or residual stimuli of the situation. When these stimuli in total fall outside of the client's adaptive zone, maladaptation is occurring and a nursing diagnosis is made. Manipulation of the focal and contextual stimuli is the goal of nursing implementation, so the client's adaptation can occur.

NOTES

1. Callista Roy, *Introduction to Nursing: An Adaptation Model* (Englewood Cliffs, N.J.: Prentice-Hall, Inc., 1976).
2. Ibid., p. 11.
3. Martha E. Rogers, *The Theoretical Basis of Nursing* (Philadelphia: F. A. Davis Co., 1970), pp. 47–73.
4. Roy, *An Adaptation Model*, p. 11.
5. Halbert L. Dunn, *High Level Wellness* (Va.: R. W. Beatty, Ltd., 1971), p. 2.
6. Roy, *An Adaptation Model*, p. 11.
7. Ibid., p. 18.
8. Harry Helson, *Adaptation Level Theory* (New York: Harper and Row Publishers, Inc., 1964); and Roy, *An Adaptation Model*, p. 13.
9. Alvin Toffler, *Future Shock* (New York: Bantam Books, 1970), pp. 337–342.
10. Roy, *An Adaptation Model*, p. 13.
11. Ibid.
12. Ibid., p. 14.
13. Imogene M. King, *Toward a Theory for Nursing: General Concepts of Human Behavior* (New York: John Wiley & Sons, Inc., 1971), p. 80.

14. René Dubos, *So Human an Animal* (New York: Charles Scribner's Sons, 1968), p. 167.
15. Roy, *An Adaptation Model*, pp. 15–16.
16. Ibid., p. 16.
17. Dunn, *High Level Wellness*, p. 163.
18. King, *Toward a Theory for Nursing*, p. 80.
19. Roy, *An Adaptation Model*, p. 15.
20. Ibid., p. 14.
21. Talcott Parsons, "The Position of Identity in the General Theory of Action," in *The Self in Social Interaction*, eds. Chad Gordon and Kenneth J. Gergen (New York: John Wiley & Sons, Inc., 1968), p. 20.
22. Arthur Coombs and Donald Snygg, *Individual-Behavior–A Perceptual Approach to Behavior* (New York: Harper and Row Publishers, Inc., 1959); and Marie J. Driever, *Theory of Self-Concept*, Callista Roy, ed. (Englewood Cliffs, N.J.: Prentice-Hall, Inc., 1976), pp. 180–189.
23. Ibid., pp. 192–196.
24. C. H. Anderson, *Toward a New Sociology: A Critical View* (Homewood, Ill.: The Dorsey Press, 1971), p. 1.
25. Roy, *An Adaptation Model*, p. 16.
26. Paul Watzlavick, Janet Helmick, and Don D. Jackson, *Pragmatics of Human Communication: A Study of Interactional Patterns, Pathologies and Paradoxes* (New York: W. W. Norton & Company, Inc., 1967), pp. 84–86.
27. Jay Haley, *Strategies of Psychotherapy* (New York: Grune and Stratton, Inc., 1963), p. 160.
28. Roy, *An Adaptation Model*, p. 16.
29. Ibid.
30. Walter Kempler, *Principles of Gestalt Family Therapy* (Salt Lake City, Utah: Desert Press, 1974), pp. 64–65.
31. Gerald Zuk and Ivan Boszormenyi-Nagy, *Family Therapy and Disturbed Families* (Palo Alto, Calif.: Science and Behavior Books, Inc., 1967), pp. 67–71.
32. Roy, *An Adaptation Model*, p. 29.
33. Ibid.
34. Ibid.
35. Ibid., pp. 30–33.
36. Florence Nightingale, *Notes on Nursing* (New York: Dover Publications, Inc., 1969).
37. Roy, *An Adaptation Model*, p. 36.
38. Ibid., p. 37.

15

NURSING THEORIES
AND THE NURSING PROCESS

Marjorie Stanton

In this chapter we will focus on the professional nurse's use of nursing theories/concepts as a framework for the nursing process. As professional nurses, we need to test those that we believe useful to practice. If nurses deliberately use the same theories/concepts in a variety of nursing situations, then it becomes possible to analyze the results and contribute to the body of nursing knowledge.

It is possible that a combination of these theories/concepts may be used so that the practicing nurse can identify new relationships and new ideas for testing. It is also possible that as we consistently use nursing theories/concepts in practice, we can identify those that we as professionals feel most confident with. We may also find that certain ones work better in selected situations than others. By keeping accurate records and communicating our successes and failures to others, the practice of nursing becomes more scientific and rational.

Using various nursing theories/concepts, the focus of nursing practice will differ. Florence Nightingale focused on changing and manipulating the environment in order to put the patient in the best possible conditions for nature to act. She also emphasized the point that nurses should alleviate and prevent unnecessary suffering and pain. Nightingale's notions about nursing laid the groundwork for and influenced other nursing theorists (see Chapter 3).

Virginia Henderson views nursing as doing for patients what they cannot do for themselves, and she identified fourteen components of nursing care that need to be considered (see Chapter 5). Her view of nursing seems to foster dependence initially, although her goal is to make the patient independent. The influence of Henderson is seen in the writings of later nursing theorists.

Faye Abdellah focused on the nurse rather than on the patient. She provided a means for categorizing patient needs under twenty-one common nursing problems relative to caring for patients (see Chapter 8). There is some similarity to Henderson's fourteen components of basic nursing care.

Hildegard Peplau presents nursing as therapeutic interactions between the nurse and patient in order to clarify the patient's problems and to set mutually acceptable goals to solving those problems. Conflict may occur if the nurse and patient cannot come to agreement about the goals; however, both the patient and nurse should grow from this experience (see Chapter 6). Peplau identified four phases in the relationship: orientation, identification, exploration, and resolution. Her influence on the notion of nursing as interpersonal in nature is pervasive.

Ida Jean Orlando advances to some extent Henderson's theory of nursing since she believes that the nurse helps patients meet a perceived need that the patients cannot meet for themselves. She fosters the dependency relationship as does Henderson, but stresses the interaction between the nurse and patient and the advocacy role of the nurse. Orlando believes that nurses care only for ill people and it is the physician who identifies the patients' illness. She believes that nursing is a deliberative action (see Chapter 9).

Ernestine Wiedenbach strongly believes that the nurse's individual philosophy lends credence to nursing care. She believes that nurses help to meet the needs that the individual identifies as the experienced need for help. Wiedenbach also believes nursing to be a deliberative action, as does Orlando (see Chapter 10).

Martha Rogers developed the principles of homeodynamics, which focus on the wholeness of man and man's interaction with his environment. The movement of man toward maximum health is the purpose of nursing. Rogers believes that the science of nursing is the science of man (see Chapter 12).

Lydia Hall's notion of nursing centers around three components: care, core, and cure. Care represents nurturance and is exclusive to nursing. Core involves the therapeutic use of self and emphasizes the use of reflection. Cure focuses on nursing related to the physician's orders. Hall views the three components as interrelated with one component taking precedence over the other two at varying points during the patient's course of progress. Hall's focus is primarily on the ill adult during the recovery stage (see Chapter 4).

Dorothea Orem focuses on the individual and his or her need for self-care action and identifies this action as universal self-care, that which meets basic human needs, or as health deviation self-care, that which relates to needs acquired in the event of illness, injury, or disease. Orem identifies three types of nursing systems: wholly compensatory, partly compensatory, and supportive-educative. Orem's system of nursing is similar in nature to Henderson's general concepts of nursing (see Chapter 7).

Myra Levine sees nursing as human interaction: the dependency of individuals on one another. She uses four conservation principles to describe nursing interventions: conservation of energy, conservation of structural integrity, conservation of personal integrity, and conservation of social integrity. She believe this provides a way to view people holistically. Levine uses the concept of organismic response to illness, which indicates to what extent adaptation is taking place (see Chapter 11).

Callista Roy's major emphasis is on the individual's ability to adapt in situations of health and illness—adaptation nursing. Each person is viewed as a biopsychosocial being with differing ways of adapting to an ever-changing environment. She uses the health-illness continuum as a way of identifying where the individual falls on the scale between death and peak wellness. Roy also uses the concepts of biological integrity, psychological integrity, and social integrity, which are similar to Levine's conservation principles (see Chapter 14).

Imogene King views man as the central focus of nursing. She looks at the concepts of social systems, perceptions, interpersonal relations, and health, and their impact on man. She considers man to be a reacting, time-oriented, social being. All these factors imply a relationship and adaptiveness to and with the environment. Man is the central focus of nursing and nursing is a process of action, reaction, interaction, and transaction (see Chapter 13).

A review of the theories presented indicates that there are similarities and differences among them. All the theorists were influenced by each other in their advancement of nursing knowledge. This fact is valuable and useful to the students of professional nursing practice. The concept of looking specifically at the environment in relationship to patients/clients was initiated by Nightingale and was considered later by King, Orem, Roy, and Rogers; but was not specifically considered by Henderson, Abdellah, Peplau, and Orlando. The concept of dependency and its role in nursing was identified by Henderson and used by Orlando, Orem, and Levine; but independence is fostered by the theories/concepts of Peplau, Rogers, Hall, and King. Adaptation is considered in the theories/concepts of Nightingale, King, Levine, Rogers, and Roy; however, where Roy views adaptation as health-producing, Rogers's concept of adaptation would be viewed as not being conducive to health. Peplau, Levine, and King emphasize interpersonal/interactive concepts in their writings, although these concepts are not overlooked by other theorists, e.g., Hall and Orlando. The theories/concepts of Henderson, Orlando, Hall, Orem, and Levine seem primarily useful in the care of the ill, whereas those of Nightingale, Peplau, Wiedenbach, King, Rogers, and Roy are useful for caring for the well and the ill. Abdellah's ideas seem more consistent with the technical aspects of nursing care, whereas the others' ideas do not.

One way of looking at the differences among the nurse theorists is to explore the variety of ways they characterized nursing actions. A quick summary of the theorists presented identifies at least three different forms of nursing actions: (1) assuming responsibility for the person until he/she is ready to assume responsibility for self; (2) changing or manipulating the environment to facilitate health and (3) helping the person toward some goal. The reader may be able to identify other similarities and differences.

The practitioners of nursing need to use those theories/concepts that are most useful in a given situation. As stated earlier, a combination of theories/concepts can be considered and if used consistently should be analyzed by the user as to their effectiveness. By using various nursing theories/concepts, the focus and consequences of nursing practice may differ.

Let us consider the following situation: Mrs. Mary James is a sixty-eight-year-old woman recovering from a stroke that occurred three days ago. She has weakness of the left side of her body. She is left-handed and requires retraining in the following areas: balancing while standing, climbing stairs, self-feeding, bladder control, and personal hygiene activities including dressing. She is in a hospital room with four other patients and is in the bed nearest the door. There is one window in the room. Before her hospitalization for the stroke, Mrs. James maintained her own home, was quite independent, volunteered one day a week at the local hospital, and was active in the local garden club.

Table 15-1 provides a brief overview of the direction a nurse might take using three of the nursing theories as a framework for the nursing process. You will note that although each theorist moves the patient to some point of independence, the methods are different due to different orientations. Nightingale focuses more on manipulation of environment, whereas Orlando and Hall focus more on patient/nurse interaction. The nature of the interaction is particular to the theorist. Hall definitely uses the technique of reflection; Orlando looks at how the nurse's behavior may affect the patient. A fully developed nursing process using any one of the theories as a framework would provide much more detailed and specific information about the patient. The brief overview gives the reader an idea of how the process might differ if a particular theory were used. It is not intended to be an all-inclusive discussion on nursing care for Mrs. James.

The consistent use of selected nursing theories/concepts in nursing practice provides a way to validate and test these theories/concepts. The transmission of such knowledge by practicing nurses and nurse researchers adds to the unique body of knowledge necessary to a profession.

The systematic use of nursing theories/concepts provides a structure and discipline for nursing practice. It also provides a framework for teaching professional nursing students how to base practice on knowledge.

Table 15-1

Overview of Theories/Concepts and Nursing Process

Theorist	Assessment	Nursing Diagnosis	Planning	Implementation	Evaluation
Nightingale	Focus on environment of patient. What in environment is contributing to disability or illness of patient? What are inhibiting factors, i.e., position of bedside table; lack of flowers; too far from window; slippery, cold floor; lack of space (four-bed room); too many people in room?	Related to environment or what is lacking in the environment as a condition to restore health, i.e., crowded, restricted environment that inhibits movement toward independence and health.	Focus is on identifying those areas of the environment needing modification or change to provide the patient with the best possible conditions for nature to restore or improve health; i.e., remove restrictions, maximize use of right hand, provide sunlight and ventilation, etc.	Carries out the actions necessary to change or manipulate the environment to provide optimum conditions for restoration or improvement of health. Move to room with two beds for more space but with companionship; provide chair near the window; place bedside table & things needed by patient on right side of bed; provide warm, sturdy slippers or shoes; place other patient in room on right side of patient; provide flowers.	Relative to how well the changes of or manipulating in the environment worked to effect optimal conditions for restoration or improvement of health, i.e., able to move about room with some assistance. Sits by window and talks to patient in room. Uses right hand to feed self and care for other needs. Arranges flowers in room. Taking an interest in what is happening inside and outside the room.
Orlando	Focus on collecting data relative to the immediate situation; i.e., Mrs. James has left side weakness.	Relates to identifying the patient's needs that patient cannot meet by self. This is validated with the	Focus is on planning with patient & mutually setting goals; i.e., clarifying with Mrs. James that she	Carries out the nursing activities necessary to meet Mrs. James' needs; i.e., assisting Mrs.	Related to Mrs. James's behavior in terms of feeding and bathing herself using the right

Theorist	Assessment	Nursing Diagnosis	Planning	Implementation	Evaluation
	What are the factors identified in this situation, i.e., inability to feed self, difficulty in bathing self, difficulty in balancing? The nurse also clarifies own reaction to the patient's behavior; i.e., "This patient is going to need a lot of help initially. Can I handle it?"	client; i.e., Mrs. James needs to be taught to use her right hand to feed and bathe self.	indeed needs to learn to use her right hand in order to feed and bathe self.	James to use her right hand to eat—do not feed patient, place bedside table on right side of patient, teach patient to stand and move without assistance.	hand. Also looks at how well nurse functioned. Uses right hand to eat but needs encouragement. Able to get out of bed with assistance, can walk to bathroom, able to dress self with assistance—"I (nurse) was able to move patient to this point."
Hall	Focus on increasing Mrs. James's self-awareness through observation and reflection. Helps Mrs. James hear herself; i.e., "I'm a sick woman. I can't take care of myself. I can't even dress or feed myself. Everyone is looking at me." Biological data are also being collected; i.e., cannot grasp or hold with left hand.	Statement of the patient's need or problem. The patient is in control; i.e., "I need to learn to take care of myself. I need to learn to use my right hand to feed and dress myself. I need to think about myself for awhile and not worry about others."	Focus is on setting goals and priorities with patient; i.e., needs to learn to care for self: 1. Learn to use right hand to feed and dress self. 2. Walk by self to bathroom. 3. Improve self-concept.	Carries out plans with the patient. Intimate bodily care is given; i.e., help patient to feed self and begin to let patient use right hand. Assist patient to dress until she learns to dress self. Support and listen to patient.	Related to patient's progress toward goals; i.e., able to feed self with right hand, able to dress self with assistance, able to walk to bathroom with assistance, able to state, "I think I'll be able to take care of myself."

GLOSSARY

Adaptation (Levine)* Process of adjusting or modifying behavior or functioning to fit the situation.

Adaptation (Rogers) Change resulting from the interaction of man and his environment. The change occurs as an ongoing evolving process that can never return to the original state.

Adaptation (Roy) Positive response to internal or external change using biopsychosocial mechanisms.

Adaptation level (Roy) Condition of the person, or the individual's range of coping ability.

Automatic activities (Orlando) Nursing actions decided on for reasons other than the patient's immediate need.

Care (Hall) The exclusive aspect of nursing that provides the patient bodily comfort through "laying on of hands" and provides an opportunity for closeness.

Complementarity (Rogers) The continuous, mutual, simultaneous interaction process between human and environmental fields.

Concept An abstract notion; a vehicle of thought that involves images; an element used to develop theories.

*When a term relates specifically to a theorist, the name of the theorist appears in parentheses after the term.

Conceptual framework Group of interrelated concepts.

Conservation (Levine) To keep together or maintain a proper balance.

Conservation of energy (Levine) Balancing energy output with energy input to avoid excessive fatigue.

Conservation of personal integrity (Levine) Maintenance or restoration of the patient's sense of identity and self-worth.

Conservation of social integrity (Levine) Acknowledgement of the patient as a social being.

Conservation of structural integrity (Levine) Refers to maintaining or restoring the structure of the body.

Contextual stimuli (Roy) Stimuli of the person's internal or external world, other than the environmental change, that influence the situation and are measurable or reportable by the person.

Core (Hall) The shared aspect with any health professional who therapeutically uses a freely offered closeness to help the patient discover who he is.

Covert problem Hidden or concealed condition.

Culture (Rogers) The integrated pattern of human behavior that includes thought, speech, action, and artifacts, and depends on man's capacity for learning and transmitting knowledge to succeeding generations.

Cure (Hall) An aspect shared with medical personnel in which the nurse helps the patient and family through medical, surgical, and/or rehabilitative care.

Deliberative actions (Orlando) Nursing actions that ascertain or meet the patient's immediate need.

Environment (Nightingale) External conditions and influences that affect life and development.

Equifinality An open system may attain a time-independent state independent of initial conditions and determined only by the system parameters.

Exploitation phase (Peplau) The third phase of Peplau's nurse-patient relationship. The patient takes full advantage of all available services while feeling an integral part of the helping environment. Goals are met through a collaborative effort as the patient becomes independent during convalescence.

Focal stimulus (Roy) Environmental change.

General systems theory A general science of wholeness.

Goal The end stated in broad terms toward whatever effort is directed.

Health (Abdellah) Dynamic state of human functioning whereby the individual continually adapts to internal and external stresses in an attempt to achieve maximum potential for daily living.

Health deviation self-care (Orem) All those demands required in the event of illness, injury, or disease.

Helicy (Rogers) The nature and direction of human and environmental change; change that is continuously innovative, probabilistic, and characterized by increasing diversity of the human field and environmental field pattern and organization emerging out of the continuous, mutual, simultaneous interaction between the human and environmental fields and manifesting nonrepeating rhythmicities.

Holism A theory that the universe and especially living nature is correctly seen in terms of interacting wholes that are more than the mere sum of elementary particles.

Homeodynamics (Rogers) A way of viewing man in his wholeness. Changes in the life process of man are irreversible, nonrepeatable, rhythmical in nature, and evidence growing complexity of pattern and organization. Change proceeds by continuous repatterning of both man and environment by resonating waves, and reflects the mutual simultaneous interaction between the two at any given point in space-time.

Humanism (Rogers) A doctrine, attitude, or way of life centered on human interests or values. A philosophy that asserts the dignity and worth of man and his capacity for self-realization through reason, and that often rejects supernaturalism.

Identification phase (Peplau) The second phase of Peplau's nurse-patient relationship. The perceptions and expectations of the patient and nurse become more involved while building a working relationship of further identifying the problem and deciding on appropriate plans for improved health maintenance.

Illness (Levine) State of altered health.

Interpersonal relationships (King) Interaction of two or more for a purpose over a period of time.

Need (Orlando) A requirement of the patient that, if supplied, relieves or diminishes his immediate distress or improves his immediate sense of well-being.

Negentropy Open systems have mechanisms that can slow down or arrest the process of movement toward less efficiency and growth.

Nursing care plan A written guide or scheme prepared by the professional nurse that gives direction to nursing actions.

Nursing interventions (Levine) Nursing activities.

Nursing problem (Abdellah) A condition presented by a client or family that the nurse can assist him or them to solve through the performance of professional functions.

Nursing process A deliberate, intellectual activity whereby the practice of nursing is approached in an orderly, systematic manner. It includes the following components:

Assessment The process of data collection that results in a conclusion or nursing diagnosis.

Diagnosis A statement describing the client's current or potential problems or deficits.

Planning The determination of what can be done to assist the client, including setting goals, judging priorities, and designing methods to resolve problems.

Implementation Action initiated to accomplish defined goals.

Evaluation The appraisal of the client's behavioral changes due to the action of the nurse.

Nurturer (Hall) A fosterer of learning, growing, and healing.

Objective A specific means by which one proposes to accomplish or attain the goal.

Organismic response (Levine) Changes in behavior or in the level of bodily functioning.

Orientation phase (Peplau) The first phase of Peplau's nurse-patient relationship. Through assessment the patient's health needs, expectations, and goals are explored and a care plan is devised. Concurrently, the roles of nurse and patient are being identified and clarified.

Overt problem Apparent or obvious condition.

Partly compensatory system (Orem) A situation where both nurse and patient perform care measures or other actions involving manipulative tasks or ambulation.

Philosophy A statement of beliefs; a viewpoint.

Potential comforter (Hall) The role of the nurse seen by the patient during the care aspect of nursing.

Potential painer (Hall) The role of the nurse seen by the patient during the cure aspect of nursing.

Prescriptive theory (Wiedenbach) A theory that conceptualizes both the desired situation and the activities to be used to bring about that desired situation.

Problem-solving process Identifying the problem, selecting pertinent data, formulating hypotheses, testing hypotheses through the collection of data, and revising hypotheses.

Reassessment The process of collecting additional data during the planning, implementing, and/or evaluation phases of the nursing process that may lead to immediate changes in those phases, or a change in the nursing diagnosis.

Reflective technique (Hall)   The process of helping the patient see who he is by mirroring what the person's behavior says, both verbally and nonverbally.

Residual stimuli (Roy)   Characteristics of the individual that are relevant to the situation but are difficult to measure objectively.

Resolution phase (Peplau)   The fourth and final phase of Peplau's nurse-patient relationship. This phase evolves from the successful completion of the previous phases. The patient and nurse terminate their therapeutic relationship as the patient's needs are met and movement is made toward new goals.

Resonancy (Rogers)   The identification of the human field and the environmental field by wave pattern and organization manifesting continuous change from lower frequency longer waves to higher frequency shorter waves.

Self-care (Orem)   Practice of activities that individuals personally initiate and perform on their own behalf to maintain life, health, and well-being.

Supportive-educative system (Orem)   A situation where the patient is able to perform or can and should learn to perform required measures of externally or internally orientated therapeutic self-care but cannot do so without assistance.

Supportive intervention (Levine)   Action that maintains the patient's present state of altered health.

Synergistic wholeness (Rogers)   Cooperative action of discrete agencies such that the total effect is greater than the sum of the effects taken independently.

Therapeutic interpersonal relationship (Peplau)   A relationship between patient and nurse in which their collaborative effort is directed toward identifying, exploring, and resolving the patient's need productively. The relationship progresses along a continuum as each experiences growth through a greater understanding of one another's roles, attitudes, and perceptions.

Therapeutic intervention (Levine)   Action that promotes healing and restoration of health.

Theory   A way of relating concepts through the use of definitions that assists in developing significant interrelationships to describe or clarify approaches to practice.

Universal self-care (Orem)   All demands referred to as activities of daily living or those that meet basic human needs.

Wholly compensatory nursing system (Orem)   A situation in which the patient has no active role in the performance of self-care.

INDEX